MY PERSONAL PUREE COOKBOOK FOR BEGINNERS

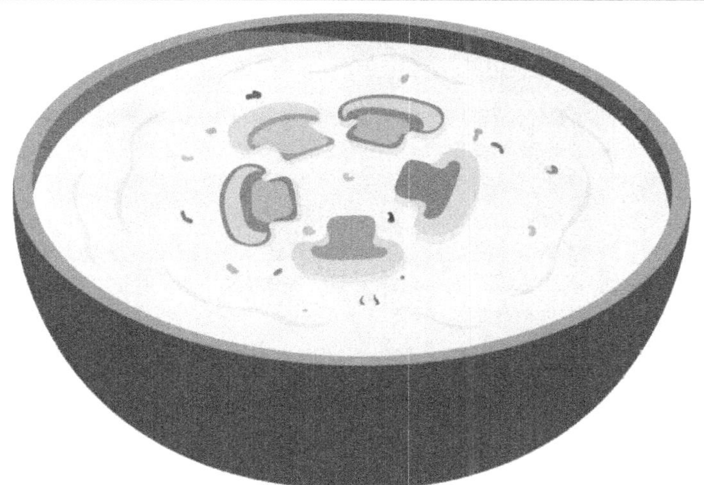

Delicious, Easy-to-Prepare Recipes Designed to Support Individuals Living with Dysphagia and Improve Swallowing difficulty

Chef Blackwood

Disclaimer

The information and recipes in this book are intended for educational and informational purposes only. The content is based on research and personal experience but does not substitute for professional medical advice. Always consult with a healthcare provider before making significant changes to your diet, especially if you have specific health conditions or concerns.

The author and publisher do not assume any responsibility for errors or omissions, or any adverse effects resulting from the use or application of any information or recipes contained in this book. The recipes are provided with the understanding that the author is not rendering medical, nutritional, or dietary advice.

TABLE OF CONTENTS

Introduction

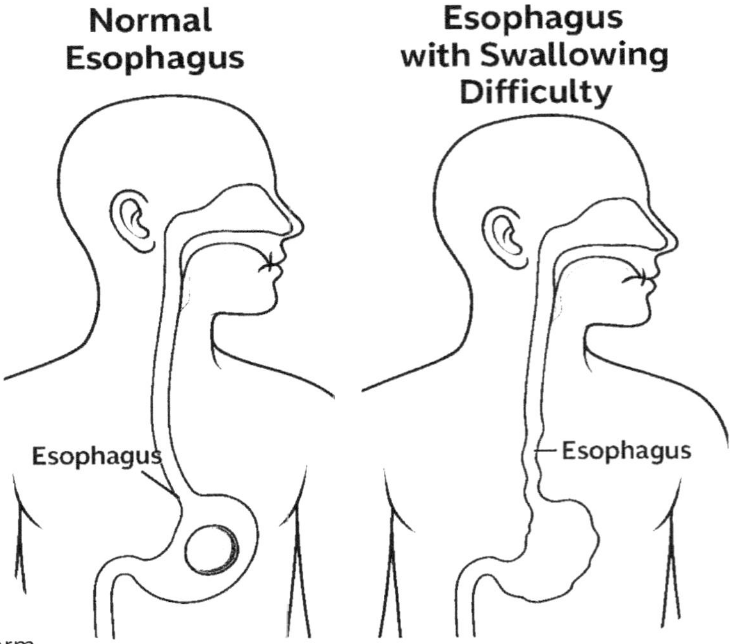

In a world where food is often celebrated for its vibrant colors, tantalizing aromas, and complex textures, being limited to pureed meals can feel like a silent struggle-one that many face but few openly discuss. It might not sound very scrumptious, but pureed meals don't have to be gross. In fact, the overall taste is largely dependent on the texture of the meal. If you're going to eat pureed meals, you'd better know how to make it delicious, and that includes creating the right texture. Your ingredients should be smooth, not chunky. All chunky ingredients can really throw the texture of the puree out of whack, causing it to be quite repulsive. Instead, opt for smooth apple sauces and creamy soups.

Normal Esophagus

Esophagus with Swallowing Difficulty

Esophagus

Esophagus

Imagine the frustration of watching a loved one push away their food, not because they are not hungry, but because the texture is off, the flavor is bland, or the meal simply looks unappetizing. This book is born from that very empathy-a heartfelt mission to transform pureed meals from a source of dread into an experience of comfort, nourishment, and even delight. Whether you are caring for an infant just beginning solids, supporting an elderly parent with swallowing difficulties, or managing a medical condition that requires texture-modified diets, this book is your comprehensive guide to making pureed meals that are as appealing as they are nutritious.

We understand that pureed food preparation is not just about blending ingredients; it's about restoring dignity and joy to every bite. A proper food processor is your best ally here. While a blender can do the job, food processors excel at creating the ideal texture and consistency, ensuring your purees are silky smooth and inviting. Plus, a large food processor allows you to prepare bulk meals to store for later, saving precious time and effort. Hospitals often use molds to shape pureed meals into solid-looking dishes, making them visually appealing and less intimidating. It's really mind over matter, so give molds a shot if your loved one is having difficulty with their meals.

This book goes beyond mere recipes. It is a celebration of texture and flavor, a practical manual filled with expert tips, from choosing the right ingredients and seasoning to mastering cooking techniques that preserve nutrients and enhance taste. You will find recipes that cater to diverse dietary needs-dairy-free, gluten-free, nut-free, soy-free, egg-free, low-sodium, sugar-free, vegan, and more-because everyone deserves to enjoy their food without compromise.

Every chapter is crafted to empower you with knowledge and confidence. You'll learn how to progress textures safely and effectively, how to enrich meals with natural herbs and spices, and how to present pureed foods in ways that stimulate appetite and pleasure. This is not just about survival; it's about thriving with pureed meals that nourish the body and soul.

If you've ever felt overwhelmed or uninspired by the prospect of pureed diets, this book will change your perspective. It invites you to embrace creativity, compassion, and culinary skill to transform what might seem like a limitation into an opportunity for care and connection. Because food is more than fuel-its love made visible, and even in pureed form, it can be delicious, comforting, and beautiful.

Dive in and discover how pureed meals can become a source of joy, health, and togetherness. Your journey to mastering the art of pureed cooking starts here.

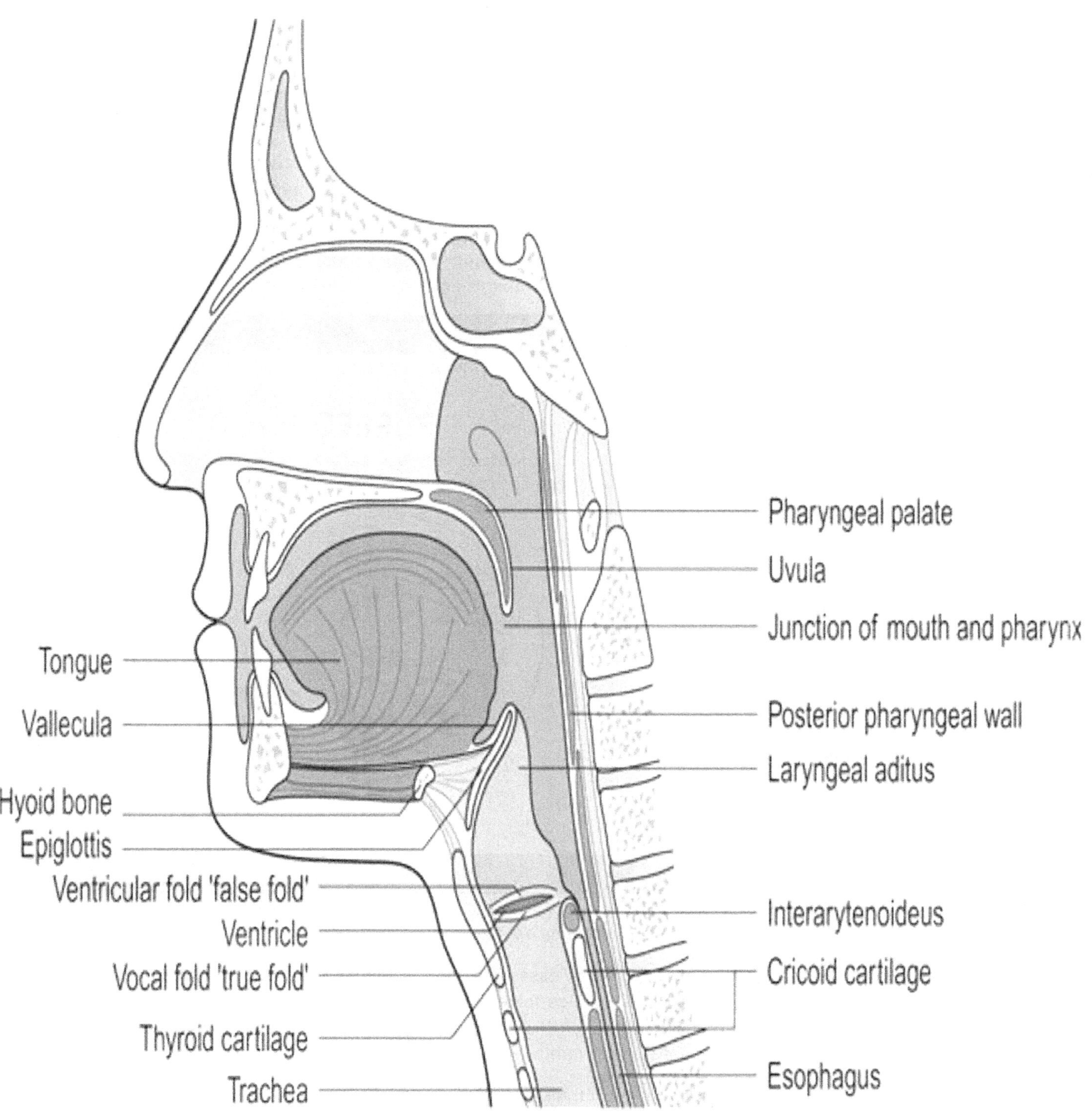
Pharyngeal palate
Uvula
Junction of mouth and pharynx
Tongue
Posterior pharyngeal wall
Vallecula
Laryngeal aditus
Hyoid bone
Epiglottis
Ventricular fold 'false fold'
Interarytenoideus
Ventricle
Vocal fold 'true fold'
Cricoid cartilage
Thyroid cartilage
Esophagus
Trachea

Chapter 1

Understanding Pureed Foods

What Are Pureed Foods?

Pureed foods are solid foods that have been blended or processed into a smooth, pudding-like texture with no lumps, making them easy to swallow without chewing. This texture modification is important for people who have difficulty chewing or swallowing due to medical conditions or treatments. Pureeing food involves chopping it into small pieces, cooking it until tender, and then blending it with liquids such as broth, juice, milk, or water to achieve the right consistency. The goal is to create a smooth, cohesive food that is safe and comfortable to eat, often resembling baby food in texture. Pureed foods can include a wide variety of items like fruits, vegetables, meats, dairy, and grains, as long as they can be transformed into this uniform, soft texture

Who Needs a Pureed Diet?

A pureed diet is typically recommended for individuals who have difficulty chewing or swallowing solid foods safely, a condition known as dysphagia. This includes people with medical conditions such as stroke, Parkinson's disease, multiple sclerosis, head, or neck cancers, or those recovering from surgery or radiation affecting the mouth, throat, or jaw. It is also advised for individuals with dental problems like missing teeth, painful gums, or ill-fitting dentures that make chewing difficult or uncomfortable. Children who are developing their chewing skills may also benefit from pureed foods. Additionally, some people with gastrointestinal issues like gastroparesis or neurodiverse conditions such as autism spectrum disorder may require pureed diets to ensure safe and adequate nutrition. Pureed foods help reduce the risk of choking and aspiration by providing a smooth, cohesive texture that requires no chewing and is easier to swallow and digest

PUREED FOOD

Pureed food is any food that has been blended, processed, or strained to a smooth, cohesive texture without lumps or chunks.

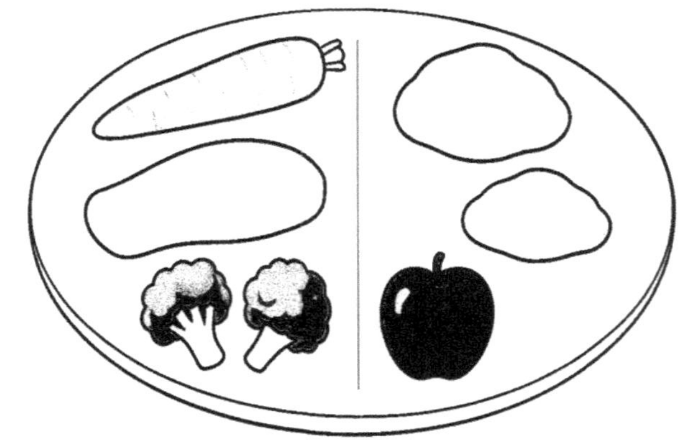

The Medical Context

Working with healthcare professionals is essential when managing a pureed diet, especially for individuals with swallowing difficulties or other medical conditions affecting eating.

Speech and Language Therapists (SLTs) play a key role by assessing and diagnosing swallowing problems (dysphagia). They determine the safest food and liquid consistencies for each individual, including whether pureed foods are necessary and if additional modifications like sieving or thickening liquids are required. SLTs provide strategies and techniques to make eating and drinking as safe, comfortable, and enjoyable as possible.

Dietitians collaborate closely with patients to ensure their pureed diet is nutritionally adequate and balanced. They offer practical advice on incorporating nutrient-rich and fiber-rich foods into pureed meals, suggest ways to fortify foods for extra calories or protein, and help plan meals that meet individual dietary needs and preferences. Dietitians also guide food choices to avoid and how to maintain hydration while following texture-modified diets.

Doctors and Other Healthcare Providers oversee the overall medical management, addressing underlying conditions that contribute to swallowing difficulties. They coordinate care among specialists and monitor complications such as weight loss, dehydration, or nutritional deficiencies that may arise from altered diets.

Effective communication among these professionals ensures that pureed diets are tailored safely to the individual's needs, optimizing nutrition, safety, and quality of life. Patients and caregivers are encouraged to follow professional guidance closely and ask questions to clarify any concerns about diet preparation, consistency, or nutritional adequacy

Benefits, Challenges, and Common Misconceptions

Benefits of Pureed Foods

The primary benefit of pureed foods is their smooth, lump-free texture, which makes them much easier to swallow and digest compared to solid foods. This is especially crucial for individuals with dysphagia or other swallowing difficulties, as pureed foods reduce the risk of choking and aspiration pneumonia-a serious lung infection caused by food or liquid entering the airway. By minimizing these risks, pureed diets provide a safer way to consume essential nutrients.

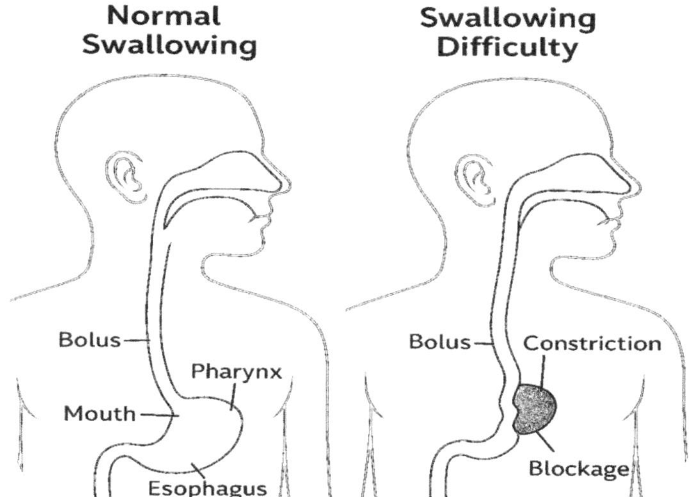

Pureed foods also help maintain adequate nutrition and hydration. For people who struggle to chew or swallow, eating solid food can be exhausting or painful, leading to reduced food intake, weight loss, and malnutrition. Pureed meals, being easier to consume, encourage sufficient calorie and nutrient intake, supporting muscle strength, immune function, and overall health. Additionally, pureed foods can be thinned with liquids like broth or milk to increase fluid intake, helping prevent dehydration, which is common among elderly or medically compromised individuals.

Another benefit is the flexibility pureed diets offer. Many foods-vegetables, fruits, meats, grains, and dairy-can be transformed into purees, allowing individuals to enjoy a variety of flavors and maintain a balanced diet. With creative preparation and seasoning, pureed meals can be both nutritious and enjoyable, improving quality of life for those affected.

Challenges of Pureed Foods

Despite these benefits, pureed diets come with challenges. One major issue is the potential for decreased appetite and food enjoyment. The texture and appearance of pureed food can be unappealing or monotonous, leading to reduced interest in eating and possible nutritional deficits. This emotional and sensory impact can affect mental well-being and social interactions around meals.

Preparing pureed foods can also be time-consuming and labor-intensive, especially when aiming for nutritious, flavorful, and visually appealing meals. Achieving the right consistency-smooth, cohesive, and moist without being too thin or sticky-requires skills and sometimes specialized equipment. Additionally, pureed foods may have a shorter shelf life and require careful storage and reheating to maintain safety and quality.

Another challenge is ensuring nutritional adequacy. Some pureed foods may lose fiber or certain nutrients during processing, and it can be harder to incorporate enough protein, calories, and variety without careful planning. Working with dietitians is often necessary to tailor pureed diets to individual needs.

Common Misconceptions About Pureed Foods

There are several misconceptions that can create hesitation or misunderstanding about pureed diets:

- **Pureed Food Is Only for the Elderly or Seriously Ill:** While common among older adults, pureed diets are prescribed for people of all ages with swallowing or chewing difficulties, including those recovering from surgery, neurological conditions, or injuries.
- **Pureed Food Is Bland and Unappetizing:** With proper seasoning, herbs, and creative presentation, pureed meals can be flavorful and visually appealing, helping to maintain appetite and enjoyment.
- **Pureed Diets Are Temporary:** For some, pureed diets are short-term during recovery, but for others with chronic conditions, they may be a long-term or permanent necessity.
- **All Pureed Foods Are the Same:** Pureed food textures vary widely and must be carefully tailored to individual swallowing abilities, often following standardized frameworks like IDDSI to ensure safety.
- **Pureed Food Is Nutritionally Inferior:** When well-planned, pureed diets can meet all nutritional requirements, including adequate calories, protein, vitamins, and minerals.

Emotional and Social Impact of Transitioning to Pureed Foods

Many people on pureed diets report feelings of frustration, loss, and diminished enjoyment related to eating. Since food is deeply connected to pleasure, identity, and independence, having to switch to pureed foods-often due to medical conditions-can be emotionally challenging. The altered texture and appearance of pureed meals can make eating less satisfying and even distressing. Studies show that patients often experience poorer meal satisfaction because pureed foods tend to have less recognizable taste and appearance, which can reduce appetite and overall food intake.

The loss of familiar food textures and the inability to identify foods by sight or taste can lead to feelings of disconnection and sadness. This emotional toll may contribute to decreased motivation to eat, risking malnutrition and weight loss. However, research also suggests that improving the taste, appearance, and recognizability of pureed foods-such as using moulded purees that resemble the original food shapes-can significantly enhance meal satisfaction and emotional well-being.

Social Impact

Eating is inherently a social activity that fosters connection, communication, and enjoyment. Transitioning to pureed foods can disrupt these social experiences. Seniors and others on pureed diets often feel isolated during meals, especially when their food looks and tastes different from what others are eating. This difference can make social dining awkward or uncomfortable, leading some to avoid sharing meals altogether.

The change in diet can also affect one's sense of dignity and normalcy. Pureed foods are sometimes perceived as "baby food" or associated with illness, which may cause embarrassment or reluctance to eat in public or with family and friends. This can contribute to social withdrawal and feelings of loneliness.

Addressing Emotional and Social Challenges

Improving the sensory appeal of pureed foods-through enhanced flavor, attractive presentation, and recognizability-can help restore some joy and dignity to eating. Caregivers and food service providers are encouraged to focus on making pureed meals flavorful and visually appealing, using techniques like moulding and seasoning to mimic regular foods.

Supporting individuals emotionally by acknowledging their feelings, involving them in meal choices, and encouraging social dining can also mitigate negative impacts. Creating a respectful and inclusive mealtime environment helps maintain social connections and improves overall quality of life.

Chapter 2

Science and Standards of Texture and Consistency

Understanding Food Textures: From Soft to Pureed

Understanding food textures-from soft to pureed-is essential for safely managing diets for individuals with chewing or swallowing difficulties. Texture modification helps ensure food is safe to swallow while maintaining nutritional value and enjoyment.

Spectrum of Food Textures

Food textures range from regular solid foods to various modified consistencies designed to meet different swallowing abilities. Key texture categories include:

- **Soft Foods:** These are tender, moist, and easy to chew foods that require minimal effort to break down. Examples include cooked vegetables, soft fruits, tender meats, and well-cooked pasta. Soft foods maintain their shape but are gentle on the teeth and gums.
- **Minced and Moist Foods:** This texture involves foods chopped into very small, uniform pieces (less than ½ cm or ¼ inch) that are moist enough to stick together, making them easier to chew and swallow. Minced foods still require some chewing but reduce the risk of choking.
- **Pureed Foods:** Pureed foods are blended to a smooth, homogeneous, pudding-like consistency with no lumps or visible particles. They are moist but thick enough to hold their shape on a spoon without separating them into liquids and solids. Pureed foods require no chewing and are usually eaten with a spoon.

Characteristics of Pureed Foods

According to established guidelines such as the International Dysphagia Diet Standardisation Initiative (IDDSI) and health services protocols:

- **Consistency:** Pureed foods should be smooth and free of lumps or stringy bits, resembling commercial pudding or mousse. The texture must be uniform, without any water separation.
- **Thickness:** They should be thick enough to mound on a spoon and hold their shape but still soft enough to fall off easily when the spoon is tilted (IDDSI Level 4).
- **Preparation:** Foods are typically cooked until very tender, then blended or processed until smooth. Liquids like broth, milk, or juice may be added gradually (about 1 tablespoon at a time) to achieve the desired moistness without making the puree runny. Straining may be used to remove skin or seeds for a finer texture.
- **Testing:** The IDDSI Fork Drip Test and Spoon Tilt Test are practical methods to ensure the puree has the correct consistency. The food should not drip continuously through a fork but may form a small tail, and it should hold shape on a spoon yet fall off easily when tilted.

Transitioning from Soft to Pureed

Soft foods require some chewing and are suitable for individuals with mild swallowing difficulties. Minced and moist foods reduce particle size to ease chewing and swallowing. Pureed foods eliminate the need to chew altogether, designed for those with more severe dysphagia or reduced tongue control.

Importance of Proper Texture Modification

Properly modified textures prevent choking, aspiration, and discomfort during eating. They also help maintain adequate nutrition and hydration by making food safer and more palatable. Texture modification must balance safety with enjoyment, as overly smooth or bland purees can reduce appetite and quality of life.

The International (IDDSI) Framework Explained

The International Dysphagia Diet Standardisation Initiative (IDDSI) Framework is a globally recognized system that provides standardized terminology and testing methods to describe food textures and drink thicknesses for individuals with swallowing difficulties (dysphagia). It consists of a continuum of eight levels, numbered 0 through 7, designed to improve safety and communication among healthcare providers, caregivers, and food service professionals worldwide.

Structure of the IDDSI Framework

- **Drink Levels (0 to 4):**
  These levels classify liquids based on their thickness, ranging from thin (Level 0) to extremely thick (Level 4). The thickness affects how easily a liquid flows and is safely swallowed.
- **Food Levels (3 to 7):**
  These levels describe food textures from liquidized (Level 3) to regular, easy-to-chew foods (Level 7). The pureed food level is Level 4, characterized by smooth, homogeneous textures that require no chewing.

Purpose and Use

The framework aims to provide a common language and clear guidelines to ensure individuals with dysphagia receive foods and drinks that match their swallowing abilities, reducing risks such as choking and aspiration. It is prescriptive rather than restrictive, encouraging offering all safe food and drink options to improve quality of life.

Testing Methods

IDDSI includes practical, standardized tests to confirm the consistency of foods and drinks under serving conditions:

- **Fork Drip Test:** Assesses whether food flows through the fork prongs, helping to determine thickness and cohesiveness for Levels 3 to 5 foods.
- **Spoon Tilt Test:** Evaluates stickiness and cohesiveness by observing how food behaves on a spoon.
- **Fork and Spoon Pressure Tests:** Measure firmness by applying pressure to food, relevant for Levels 4 to 7.
- **Finger Test:** Offers an accessible method to assess texture when other tools are unavailable.

Importance

By standardizing terminology and testing, the IDDSI Framework reduces confusion and errors in diet texture selection, which have been linked to serious adverse events. It facilitates safer care across settings and countries, supporting clinicians in making informed recommendations based on comprehensive assessments.

In summary, the IDDSI Framework is an internationally adopted, evidence-based tool that categorizes food and drink textures into eight clear levels, supported by simple tests, to improve the safety and quality of life for people with swallowing difficulties worldwide.

Using Thickeners: Natural and Commercial Options

Using thickeners is a key technique to achieve the safe and desirable consistency of pureed foods, especially for individuals with swallowing difficulties. Thickeners help create a cohesive, uniform texture that prevents the separation of liquids and solids, ensuring the food is safe to swallow and pleasant to eat. There are both natural and commercial thickening options available, each with their own advantages and considerations.

Natural Thickeners

Natural thickeners are food-based ingredients that not only improve texture but can also add nutritional value and flavor. Common natural thickeners include:

- **Pureed Beans and Legumes:** These add protein and fiber while thickening the texture.
- **Cooked and Pureed Starchy Vegetables:** Such as pumpkin, potato, sweet potato, and squash, which provide bulk and creaminess.
- **Finely Ground Crackers, Breadcrumbs, or Cereals:** These absorb moisture and add thickness without drastically changing flavor.
- **Vegetable Powders:** Dried and powdered vegetables can boost nutrition and help thicken purees naturally.

Natural thickeners are beneficial because they enhance the nutritional profile of pureed foods and often improve taste. However, they may require recipe development and testing to achieve the right texture consistently.

Commercial Thickeners

Commercial thickeners are specially formulated powders designed to thicken liquids and pureed foods quickly and reliably. They come in two main types:

- **Starch-Based Thickeners:** Made from modified starches, these powders thicken foods effectively but may continue to thicken over time and can be affected by heat or acidic foods. They are not resistant to saliva enzymes, which can thin the texture in the mouth. Examples include Thick-It® and ThickenUp®.
- **Gum-Based Thickeners (e.g., Xanthan Gum):** These are clear, tasteless, and stable, maintaining consistent thickness over time and in the presence of saliva. They work well in both hot and cold foods and liquids and do not add calories or carbohydrates. Brands include Thick & Easy® and Simply Thick®.

Specialized Thickeners for Pureed Food Molding

Some commercial thickeners, such as Food Mold Thickener or SHAPE & SERVE® Thickener, are designed specifically for molding pureed foods. They are heat, freezing, and thaw stable, allowing pureed foods to be shaped attractively without losing consistency. These thickeners have neutral taste and help maintain uniform texture, enhancing the visual appeal and dignity of pureed meals.

Choosing and Using Thickeners

- **Consistency Levels:** Thickeners help achieve IDDSI-consistent textures such as nectar-thick, honey-thick, or pudding-thick purees, depending on swallowing needs.
- **Taste and Nutritional Value:** It's important to select thickeners that do not alter flavor negatively and, when possible, add nutritional benefits.
- **Preparation Tips:** Add thickeners gradually, blend thoroughly, and test the texture using methods like the Fork Drip and Spoon Tilt tests. Adjust as needed to avoid overly thick or runny purees.
- **Stability:** Consider how the thickener behaves with heating, freezing, or storage to maintain safe texture over time.

What are some good thickening agents for pureed foods

Some good thickening agents for pureed foods include a variety of starches, gums, and natural purees that help achieve a smooth, cohesive texture without lumps or separation. Here are the main options:

Starch-Based Thickeners

- **Cornstarch**: A common, flavorless, gluten-free powder used in sauces and soups; requires making a slurry before adding to hot liquids to avoid clumping.
- **Potato starch**: Used in soups and sauces, gluten-free, colorless, odorless, and effective at binding and thickening.
- **Tapioca starch**: Extracted from cassava, slightly sweet, good for puddings and pie fillings, suitable for gluten-free recipes.
- **Arrowroot powder**: Flavorless, colorless, has twice the thickening power of flour, and works well with acidic foods.
- **Modified cornstarch**: Often used commercially for quick thickening in packaged foods.

Gum-Based Thickeners

- **Xanthan gum**: Clear, odorless, tasteless, stable (does not thicken further after reaching desired viscosity), resistant to breakdown by saliva enzymes, suitable for thickening beverages and purees.
- **Guar gum**: Used in dairy and gluten-free recipes, though less effective in highly acidic foods.
- **Locust bean gum (carob gum)**: Used in ice cream and dairy products to improve texture.

Protein-Based Thickeners

- **Gelatin**: Derived from animal collagen, used in desserts, and can thicken purees, but not suitable for vegetarians/vegans.
- **Egg yolks**: Used as thickeners in custards and sauces.

Natural Puree and Food-Based Thickeners

- **Pureed beans or legumes**: Add both thickness and nutrition to pureed foods.
- **Pureed starchy vegetables** (e.g., pumpkin, potato, squash): Can thicken soups and sauces naturally while adding flavor and nutrients.
- **Finely ground crackers, cereals, or breadcrumbs**: Used as powders to thicken purees and add texture.

Other Natural and Commercial Thickeners

- **Pectin**: A natural starch from fruit peels, used mainly in jams and jellies, vegan-friendly
- **Agar-agar**: A vegetarian gelatin substitute derived from red algae, odorless and flavorless, forms a clear gel.
- **Commercial thickening powders**: Products like Thick-It®, Thick & Easy®, ThickenUp® contain modified starches or gums designed for dysphagia diets and pureed foods; they are easy to measure, mix, and stable in hot or cold foods without lumping.

Summary Table of Common Thickening Agents for Pureed Foods

Thickener	Source	Key Properties	Notes
Cornstarch	Corn starch	Flavorless, gluten-free, needs slurry	Common kitchen thickener
Potato starch	Potato	Gluten-free, odorless, colorless	Good for soups and gluten-free cooking
Tapioca starch	Cassava	Slightly sweet, good for puddings	Gluten-free, chewy texture in baked goods
Arrowroot powder	Tropical plants	Twice thickening power of flour	Works well in acidic foods
Xanthan gum	Bacterial polysaccharide	Clear, stable, amylase-resistant	Suitable for beverages and purees
Guar gum	Guar bean	Thickens dairy and gluten-free foods	Less effective in acidic conditions
Locust bean gum	Carob tree	Improves texture in dairy products	Used in ice creams
Gelatin	Animal collagen	Forms gels, used in desserts	Not vegan/vegetarian
Egg yolks	Eggs	Thickens custards and sauces	Adds richness
Pureed beans/veg	Natural foods	Adds nutrition and thickness	Good for natural thickening
Pectin	Fruit peels	Vegan, gels jams and jellies	Used for fruit preserves
Agar-agar	Red algae	Vegan gelatin substitute	Forms clear gels
Commercial powders	Modified starch/gums	Easy to use, stable, no lumps	Designed for dysphagia and pureed diets

Chapter 3

Nutrition on a Pureed Diet

Ensuring Balanced Nutrition: Macronutrients and Micronutrients

Ensuring balanced nutrition on a pureed diet involves carefully including all essential macronutrients-carbohydrates, proteins, and fats-as well as vital micronutrients like vitamins and minerals, while adapting foods to a smooth, safe texture.

Macronutrients

- **Carbohydrates:**
  Carbohydrates provide energy and are found in pureed grains, fruits, and vegetables. Suitable options include pureed cereals (such as oatmeal, Cream of Wheat, or cornmeal), pureed bread products, mashed potatoes, and smooth fruit purees like apples or pears. Using whole grains, when possible, adds fiber, which supports digestive health. Cooking and blending vegetables and fruits until soft and smooth ensures they retain their nutrients while being safe to swallow.

- **Proteins:**
  Protein is essential for tissue repair, immune function, and muscle maintenance. On a pureed diet, protein sources include pureed meats (chicken, beef, fish), eggs, dairy products like smooth yogurt, cottage cheese, and melted cheese, as well as plant-based proteins such as pureed tofu, lentils, beans, and smooth nut butters. Incorporating these ensures adequate protein intake, which is especially important for recovery and maintaining strength.

- **Fats:**
  Healthy fats provide concentrated energy and aid in the absorption of fat-soluble vitamins. Including sources of unsaturated fats like pureed avocado, adding cream or milk to dishes, or using oils in cooking can enrich pureed meals. Dairy products like full-fat yogurt and cheese also contribute fats. These additions enhance calorie density and improve taste and mouth feel, encouraging better intake.

Micronutrients

- **Vitamins and Minerals:**
  Fruits and vegetables are primary sources of vitamins and minerals. Pureeing a variety of cooked vegetables (carrots, spinach, squash, broccoli) and fruits (apples, peaches, pears) helps preserve these nutrients while ensuring safety. It is important to avoid skins, seeds, and fibrous parts that can pose swallowing risks. Dairy and fortified plant-based milks provide calcium and vitamin D, supporting bone health.

- **Fiber:**
  Although fiber is important for digestive health, it can be challenging to include in pureed diets due to texture restrictions. Using pureed legumes, cooked vegetables, and whole grain cereals can help maintain fiber intake without compromising safety.

Practical Tips for Balanced Pureed Meals

- **Combine Food Groups:** Aim to include a source of protein, carbohydrate, and fat at each meal, along with fruits or vegetables for vitamins and minerals.

- **Enhance Flavor and Nutrient Density:** Use milk, cream, gravies, sauces, or healthy oils to improve taste and add calories without altering texture.

- **Portion Sizes:** Follow recommended portion sizes, such as three servings of milk or dairy alternatives daily and five servings of fruits and vegetables, adjusted for pureed forms.
- **Avoid Nutrient Loss:** Cook food minimally to retain nutrients before pureeing and avoid over-thinning purees which can dilute nutrient density.
- **Variety:** Rotate different foods to cover a broad spectrum of nutrients and prevent monotony.

Protein Sources: Animal and Plant Based Options

Here is an overview of protein sources suitable for pureed diets, including both animal-based and plant-based options, based on current expert guidelines and recommendations:

Animal-Based Protein Sources for Pureed Diets

- **Poultry:** Pureed chicken or turkey (skin removed) is a high-quality protein source often recommended. It should be cooked until tender and blended to a smooth consistency.
- **Fish:** Soft fish varieties such as haddock, tilapia, cod, salmon, and flounder can be pureed or mashed. Canned tuna or salmon (packed in water) is also suitable when mashed smoothly.
- **Eggs:** Scrambled eggs or pureed boiled eggs provide easily digestible protein. Egg substitutes and egg whites can also be used for variety and additional protein.
- **Dairy:** Low-fat or fat-free cottage cheese, part-skim ricotta cheese, plain yogurt, or Greek yogurt (without fruit pieces), milk (skim, 1%, or lactose-free), and cream soups made with fat-free milk are excellent protein-rich options. Melted hard cheeses like cheddar or mozzarella can be incorporated into pureed dishes.
- **Lean Meats:** Ground lean beef, pork, or turkey (93% fat-free or higher) can be cooked and pureed to provide substantial protein.

Plant-Based Protein Sources for Pureed Diets

- **Tofu:** Silken or soft tofu pureed smoothly is a versatile, high-protein, plant-based option.
- **Beans and Legumes:** Pureed fat-free refried beans, lentils, and other legumes provide protein and fiber. Smooth peanut butter or other smooth nut butters can also be added to purees or smoothies, but nuts should be avoided whole due to choking risk.
- **Meat Alternatives:** Vegetarian sausages or other plant-based protein products that can be pureed or mashed are suitable, depending on texture and ingredients.
- **Soy Products:** Light soy milk (plain or vanilla) is a good protein source and can be used in cooking or as a beverage.

Protein Intake Recommendations

- Aim for at least 60-75 grams of protein daily, divided into three protein-containing pureed meals of about ¼ to ⅓ cup each.
- Prioritize protein intake early in meals to ensure adequate consumption.
- Consider adding protein powders or supplements (e.g., Sustagen, Ensure) if dietary intake is insufficient.
- Use cooking liquids like broth or milk to blend proteins smoothly without diluting nutrient density.

Carbohydrates and Starches for Energy

Carbohydrates and starches are essential components of a pureed diet, providing the primary source of energy needed for daily activities and bodily functions. They also supply important vitamins, minerals, and fiber, contributing to overall health and digestive function.

Role of Carbohydrates and Starches

Starchy foods such as potatoes, bread, rice, pasta, and cereals are rich in complex carbohydrates, which are broken down slowly in the body to provide a steady release of energy. This sustained energy helps prevent the body from using protein as a fuel source, allowing protein to be spared for tissue repair and maintenance. Including starchy foods regularly supports balanced nutrition and helps maintain strength and vitality, especially important for those recovering from illness or managing chronic conditions.

Suitable Pureed Carbohydrate Sources

For individuals on a pureed diet, starchy foods should be cooked until incredibly soft and then blended or mashed to a smooth, lump-free consistency. Examples include:

- Mashed potatoes or whipped sweet potatoes, prepared with added milk or butter for energy and moisture.
- Pureed pasta, rice, or noodles cooked until tender and blended smooth.
- Hot cereals such as oatmeal, Cream of Wheat®, or Cream of Rice®, which can be prepared with milk and pureed if needed.
- Pureed bread products like soft rolls, pancakes, or muffins, which can be softened with milk or gravy before pureeing.

Wholegrain or wholemeal varieties are recommended, when possible, as they provide more fiber and nutrients, but they must be finely pureed and free of lumps or skins to ensure safety.

Preparation Tips

- Cook starchy foods thoroughly until it is incredibly soft to facilitate smooth pureeing.
- Add liquids such as milk, broth, or cream gradually to achieve the desired pudding-like texture without making the puree too thin.
- Avoid foods that do not blend well or contain hard bits, such as cereals with flakes or nuts.
- Incorporate starchy vegetables like carrots, squash, or parsnips as additional carbohydrate sources when pureed.

Nutritional Importance

Starchy foods should make up just over a third of the diet, according to healthy eating guidelines, ensuring sufficient energy intake. They also contribute important B vitamins and minerals. Including a variety of starchy pureed foods helps maintain balanced nutrition and supports overall health.

Healthy Fats and Sugars

Healthy fats and sugars play important roles in a balanced pureed diet, providing essential energy, flavor, and nutrients while supporting overall health.

Healthy Fats

Healthy fats, particularly unsaturated fats, are vital for energy, cell function, and the absorption of fat-soluble vitamins (A, D, E, and K). They also help repair the body and improve the taste and texture of pureed foods, making meals more enjoyable and nourishing.

Sources of Healthy Fats Suitable for Pureed Diets:

- **Avocado:** Naturally creamy and rich in monounsaturated fats, easily blended into purees for added smoothness and nutrition.
- **Vegetable Oils:** Olive oil, canola oil, peanut oil, and other plant-based oils can be incorporated into pureed dishes or drizzled over foods to increase calorie density.
- **Fish Oil:** Found in fatty fish like salmon and mackerel, fish oil provides omega-3 fatty acids beneficial for heart and brain health. Pureed fish can be a good source.
- **Nut Butters:** Smooth peanut butter or almond butter can be added to purees or smoothies, providing healthy fats and protein, but nuts should never be given whole due to choking risk.
- **Dairy Fats:** Butter, cream, full-fat yogurt, and cheese (melted and pureed) contribute saturated fats and calories, useful for those needing extra nourishment.

It is recommended to focus more on unsaturated fats (from plant oils, fish, and avocado) and limit saturated fats (from butter, cream, and fatty meats) for long-term health benefits.

Sugars

Sugars provide a quick source of energy and can improve the palatability of pureed foods, which is important for individuals with reduced appetite or altered taste sensations. Natural sugars found in fruits and dairy, as well as added sugars in moderation, can help maintain calorie intake.

Suitable Sugar Sources for Pureed Diets:

- **Natural Fruit Sugars:** Pureed fruits like apples, pears, peaches, and bananas add sweetness along with vitamins, minerals, and fiber.
- **Honey, Syrup, and Jam:** These can be stirred into pureed foods or drinks to enhance flavor and energy content, especially for those with poor appetite.
- **Sugar:** Used sparingly, sugar can be added to homemade puddings, custards, or cereals to improve taste.
- **Milk and Dairy:** Lactose in milk and yogurt provides natural sugars and contributes to energy intake.

Important Considerations

- Avoid foods that separate (e.g., ice cream) or contain lumps, seeds, or skins that pose choking risks.
- Use sugars and fats to fortify foods for individuals with poor appetite or weight loss, but avoid low-fat, low-sugar, or diet products that reduce calorie intake.
- Balance is key: incorporate healthy fats and moderate sugars to support energy needs without compromising overall nutritional quality.

Vitamins, Minerals, and Fiber from Fruits and Vegetables

Fruits and vegetables are vital sources of vitamins, minerals, and dietary fiber, all of which play essential roles in maintaining health, especially for individuals on pureed diets who need nutrient-dense, safe-to-swallow foods.

Vitamins and Minerals from Fruits and Vegetables

Fruits and vegetables provide a broad spectrum of vitamins and minerals, many with antioxidant properties that help reduce the risk of chronic diseases:

- **Vitamin A (beta-carotene):** Found in carrots, sweet potatoes, spinach, and other colorful vegetables, vitamin A supports vision, immune function, and skin health.
- **Vitamin C:** Abundant in citrus fruits, strawberries, broccoli, and bell peppers, vitamin C is important for immune support, wound healing, and antioxidant protection.
- **Vitamin E:** Present in avocados and some green leafy vegetables, vitamin E acts as an antioxidant protecting cells from damage.
- **Folate (Vitamin B9):** Found in leafy greens, asparagus, broccoli, and legumes, folate supports DNA synthesis and cardiovascular health.
- **Magnesium, Potassium, Zinc, and Phosphorus:** These minerals, found in a variety of fruits and vegetables such as bananas, spinach, and potatoes, are crucial for muscle function, bone health, and metabolic processes.

Consuming these nutrients through whole fruits and vegetables is more beneficial than supplements, as the natural food matrix enhances absorption and provides additional phytochemicals.

Dietary Fiber from Fruits and Vegetables

Fiber is a key component of fruits and vegetables that supports digestive health, helps regulate blood sugar, lowers cholesterol, and promotes satiety. There are two types:

- **Soluble Fiber:** Found in apples, pears, carrots, and oats, soluble fiber dissolves in water and helps lower blood cholesterol and glucose levels.
- **Insoluble Fiber:** Present in skins of fruits like apples and pears, as well as in vegetables like broccoli and Brussels sprouts, insoluble fiber adds bulk to stool and aids regular bowel movements.

Examples of high-fiber fruits include raspberries (3.3 g per cup), strawberries (2 g per half cup), pears, apples, bananas, and avocados (about 10 g fiber per medium fruit). Vegetables rich in fiber include broccoli, carrots, Brussels sprouts, beets, and artichokes.

Incorporating Fruits and Vegetables into Pureed Diets

For those on pureed diets, fruits and vegetables should be cooked until soft and blended to a smooth consistency to ensure safety. Removing skins, seeds, and fibrous parts helps prevent choking hazards while preserving fiber and nutrients as much as possible. Pureed fruits like applesauce, mashed bananas, or pureed berries can provide both vitamins and fiber, while pureed cooked vegetables such as carrots, squash, and broccoli offer minerals and antioxidants.

Adapting Pureed Diets for Allergies and Special Dietary Needs

Adapting pureed diets for allergies and special dietary needs such as gluten-free, low sodium, and diabetic-friendly requirements involves careful modification of ingredients, preparation methods, and nutritional balance to ensure safety, adequacy, and palatability.

Gluten-Free Pureed Diets

For individuals with gluten intolerance or celiac disease, all gluten-containing grains (wheat, barley, rye, and their derivatives) must be excluded. Pureed diets can be adapted by using naturally gluten-free ingredients such as:

- Pureed rice, potatoes, corn, quinoa, and gluten-free oats as carbohydrate sources.
- Gluten-free flours or thickeners (e.g., rice flour, cornstarch) to achieve the desired texture without gluten contamination.
- Avoid processed foods or sauces that may contain hidden gluten.
- Ensuring strict cross-contamination prevention during preparation and serving.

Low Sodium Pureed Diets

Reducing sodium intake is critical for individuals with hypertension, heart disease, or kidney conditions. To adapt pureed diets for low sodium needs:

- Use fresh or frozen vegetables and fruits rather than canned or processed varieties, which often contain added salt.
- Prepare pureed foods from scratch, seasoning with herbs, spices, lemon juice, or vinegar instead of salt.
- Avoid adding salt during cooking or at the table.
- Choose low-sodium or no-salt-added broths and stocks when thinning purees.
- Monitor and limit processed meats and cheeses that are typically high in sodium.

Diabetic-Friendly Pureed Diets

Managing blood sugar levels is essential for diabetic individuals, so pureed diets should focus on balanced carbohydrate intake with controlled sugars and fiber:

- Include complex carbohydrates with a low glycemic index, such as pureed whole grains, legumes, and non-starchy vegetables.
- Limit pureed fruits high in natural sugars; opt for lower-sugar fruits like berries or green apples in moderation.
- Avoid added sugars, syrups, and sweetened beverages in pureed foods.
- Incorporate adequate protein and healthy fats to slow glucose absorption and promote satiety.
- Monitor portion sizes and carbohydrate content carefully to maintain blood sugar control.

Chapter 4

Breakfast

Cinnamon Roll Breakfast Smoothie

Prep Time: 5 minutes | **Cooking Time:** 0 minutes | **Per Serving:** 1

Ingredients:

- 1 cup unsweetened almond milk (or milk of choice)
- 1/2 cup plain Greek yogurt
- 1/2 cup rolled oats
- 1 frozen banana
- 1 tablespoon almond butter
- 1 teaspoon ground cinnamon
- 1 teaspoon vanilla extract
- 1 teaspoon honey or maple syrup (optional)
- A pinch of nutmeg (optional)

Instructions:

1. Add all ingredients to a blender.
2. Blend on high until smooth and creamy.
3. Taste and adjust sweetness if needed by adding honey or maple syrup.
4. Pour into a glass and enjoy immediately.

Nutritional Information (per serving):
Calories: 320 | Carbohydrates: 40g | Protein: 15g | Fiber: 6g | Fat: 9g | Sodium: 100mg | Sugar: 18g | Calcium: 250mg | Iron: 1.5mg | Potassium: 550mg

Spiced Pear Oat Baby Food Puree

Prep Time: 5 minutes | **Cooking Time:** 15 minutes | **Per Serving:** 4 servings

Ingredients:

- 2 ripe pears, peeled, cored, and chopped
- 1/4 cup rolled oats
- 1/2 teaspoon ground cinnamon
- 1/4 teaspoon ground ginger
- 1 cup water or breast milk/formula

Instructions:

1. In a small saucepan, combine pears, oats, cinnamon, ginger, and water.
2. Bring to a boil, then reduce heat and simmer for 10-15 minutes until pears and oats are soft.
3. Allow to cool slightly, then puree in a blender until smooth.
4. Add more liquid if needed to reach desired consistency.
5. Serve warm or chilled.

Nutritional Information (per serving):
Calories: 90 | Carbohydrates: 20g | Protein: 2g | Fiber: 3g | Fat: 1g | Sodium: 5mg | Sugar: 12g | Calcium: 20mg | Iron: 0.3mg | Potassium: 130mg

Oats, Spinach, and Avocado Baby Food Puree

Prep Time: 5 minutes | **Cooking Time:** 10 minutes | **Per Serving:** 4 servings

Ingredients:

- 1/4 cup rolled oats
- 1 cup fresh spinach leaves, washed
- 1/2 ripe avocado
- 1 cup water or breast milk/formula

Instructions:

1. Cook oats in water over medium heat until soft, about 5-7 minutes.
2. Add spinach during the last 2 minutes of cooking to wilt.
3. Transfer oats and spinach to a blender, add avocado, and puree until smooth.
4. Add breast milk or formula to thin if necessary.
5. Serve immediately or store refrigerated.

Nutritional Information (per serving):
Calories: 110 | Carbohydrates: 15g | Protein: 3g | Fiber: 5g | Fat: 5g | Sodium: 20mg | Sugar: 1g | Calcium: 30mg | Iron: 1mg | Potassium: 250mg

Mango + Kale Baby Food Puree with Ginger

Prep Time: 5 minutes | **Cooking Time:** 10 minutes | **Per Serving:** 4 servings

Ingredients:

- 1 ripe mango, peeled and chopped
- 1 cup kale leaves, stems removed, chopped
- 1/4 teaspoon fresh ginger, grated
- 1/2 cup water or breast milk/formula

Instructions:

1. Steam kale until tender, about 5-7 minutes.
2. Place mango, steamed kale, and grated ginger in a blender.
3. Add water or breast milk/formula and puree until smooth.
4. Adjust liquid for desired consistency.
5. Serve fresh or chilled.

Nutritional Information (per serving):
Calories: 80 | Carbohydrates: 18g | Protein: 2g | Fiber: 3g | Fat: 1g | Sodium: 15mg | Sugar: 15g | Calcium: 25mg | Iron: 0.5mg | Potassium: 200mg

3 Berry + Apple Baby Food Puree

Prep Time: 5 minutes | **Cooking Time:** 10 minutes | **Per Serving:** 4 servings

Ingredients:

- 1/2 cup strawberries, hulled
- 1/2 cup blueberries
- 1/2 cup raspberries
- 1 apple, peeled, cored, and chopped
- 1/2 cup water or breast milk/formula

Instructions:

1. Steam apple pieces until soft, about 8-10 minutes.
2. Add steamed apple and berries to a blender.
3. Add water or breast milk/formula and puree until smooth.
4. Adjust liquid to achieve desired consistency.
5. Serve immediately or refrigerate.

Nutritional Information (per serving):
Calories: 70 | Carbohydrates: 17g | Protein: 1g | Fiber: 4g | Fat: 0g | Sodium: 5mg | Sugar: 12g | Calcium: 15mg | Iron: 0.3mg | Potassium: 150mg

Roasted Pear + Date Baby Food Puree

Prep Time: 10 minutes | **Cooking Time:** 25 minutes | **Per Serving:** 4 servings

Ingredients:

- 2 ripe pears, peeled, cored, and quartered
- 4 Medjool dates, pitted
- 1/2 teaspoon ground cinnamon
- 1/2 cup water or breast milk/formula

Instructions:

1. Preheat oven to 375°F (190°C).
2. Place pears and dates on a baking sheet and roast for 20-25 minutes until soft and caramelized.
3. Transfer roasted fruit to a blender, add cinnamon and water or breast milk/formula.
4. Puree until smooth, adding more liquid if needed to achieve desired consistency.
5. Serve warm or chilled.

Nutritional Information (per serving):
Calories: 100 | Carbohydrates: 26g | Protein: 1g | Fiber: 3g | Fat: 0g | Sodium: 2mg | Sugar: 22g | Calcium: 15mg | Iron: 0.3mg | Potassium: 180mg

Peach, Mango + Carrot Baby Food Puree

Prep Time: 5 minutes | **Cooking Time:** 15 minutes | **Per Serving:** 4 servings

Ingredients:

- 1 large peach, peeled and chopped
- 1 ripe mango, peeled and chopped
- 1 large carrot, peeled and chopped
- 1/2 cup water or breast milk/formula

Instructions:

1. Steam carrot until tender, about 10-12 minutes.
2. Add peach, mango, and steamed carrot to a blender.
3. Add water or breast milk/formula and puree until smooth.
4. Adjust liquid as needed.
5. Serve immediately or refrigerate.

Nutritional Information (per serving):
Calories: 85 | Carbohydrates: 21g | Protein: 1g | Fiber: 3g | Fat: 0g | Sodium: 15mg | Sugar: 18g | Calcium: 20mg | Iron: 0.4mg | Potassium: 190mg

Roasted Blueberry + Cinnamon Baby Food Puree

Prep Time: 5 minutes | **Cooking Time:** 20 minutes | **Per Serving:** 4 servings

Ingredients:

- 1 cup fresh or frozen blueberries
- 1/2 teaspoon ground cinnamon
- 1/2 cup water or breast milk/formula

Instructions:

1. Preheat oven to 375°F (190°C).
2. Spread blueberries on a baking sheet and roast for 15-20 minutes until soft and bursting.
3. Transfer roasted blueberries to a blender, add cinnamon and water or breast milk/formula.
4. Puree until smooth, adding liquid as needed.
5. Serve warm or chilled.

Nutritional Information (per serving):
Calories: 60 | Carbohydrates: 15g | Protein: 1g | Fiber: 3g | Fat: 0g | Sodium: 1mg | Sugar: 11g | Calcium: 10mg | Iron: 0.3mg | Potassium: 90mg

Roasted Banana + Apple with Cinnamon Baby Food Puree

Prep Time: 5 minutes | **Cooking Time:** 25 minutes | **Per Serving:** 4 servings

Ingredients:

- 2 ripe bananas, peeled and sliced
- 1 large apple, peeled, cored, and sliced
- 1/2 teaspoon ground cinnamon

- 1/2 cup water or breast milk/formula

Instructions:

1. Preheat oven to 375°F (190°C).
2. Place banana and apple slices on a baking sheet and roast for 20-25 minutes until soft and caramelized.
3. Transfer roasted fruit to a blender, add cinnamon and water or breast milk/formula.
4. Puree until smooth, adding more liquid if needed.
5. Serve warm or chilled.

Nutritional Information (per serving):
Calories: 110 | Carbohydrates: 28g | Protein: 1g | Fiber: 3g | Fat: 0g | Sodium: 2mg | Sugar: 20g | Calcium: 15mg | Iron: 0.3mg | Potassium: 250mg

Apple, Raspberry with Vanilla Baby Food Puree

Prep Time: 5 minutes | **Cooking Time:** 15 minutes | **Per Serving:** 4 servings

Ingredients:

- 2 apples, peeled, cored, and roughly chopped
- 1 cup raspberries, fresh or frozen
- 1/2 vanilla bean pod (or 1 teaspoon vanilla bean extract)
- 1/3 cup water

Instructions:

1. In a medium saucepan, add apples and water. Cover and heat on medium-low for 10 minutes or until apples are tender, stirring occasionally.
2. Meanwhile, split the vanilla bean pod lengthwise and scrape out the seeds with the back of a knife.
3. Add raspberries and vanilla seeds to the saucepan and heat for an additional 5 minutes, stirring occasionally.
4. Transfer all ingredients to a blender or food processor and puree until smooth, adding water in small increments if needed to reach desired consistency.

- 1 ripe mango, peeled and chopped
- 1/2 ripe avocado
- 1/2 cup plain full-fat yogurt or breast milk/formula

Instructions:

1. Place mango, avocado, and yogurt or breast milk/formula in a blender.
2. Puree until smooth and creamy.
3. Adjust consistency by adding more yogurt or breast milk/formula if needed.
4. Serve immediately or refrigerate.

Nutritional Information (per serving):
Calories: 120 | Carbohydrates: 15g | Protein: 2g | Fiber: 4g | Fat: 6g | Sodium: 30mg | Sugar: 12g | Calcium: 80mg | Iron: 0.3mg | Potassium: 300mg

Blackberry + Kale + Apple Baby Food Puree

Prep Time: 5 minutes | **Cooking Time:** 10 minutes | **Per Serving:** 4 servings

Ingredients:

- 1 cup blackberries, fresh or frozen
- 1 cup kale leaves, stems removed, chopped
- 1 apple, peeled, cored, and chopped
- 1/2 cup water or breast milk/formula

Instructions:

1. Steam kale and apple until tender, about 8-10 minutes.
2. Place steamed kale, apple, and blackberries in a blender.
3. Add water or breast milk/formula and puree until smooth.
4. Adjust liquid to desired consistency.
5. Serve immediately or refrigerate.

Nutritional Information (per serving):
Calories: 70 | Carbohydrates: 18g | Protein: 1g | Fiber: 4g | Fat: 0g | Sodium: 10mg | Sugar: 12g | Calcium: 25mg | Iron: 0.5mg | Potassium: 160mg

Apple + Mint with Cottage Cheese Baby Food Puree

Prep Time: 5 minutes | **Cooking Time:** 10 minutes | **Per Serving:** 4 servings

Ingredients:

- 2 apples, peeled, cored, and chopped
- 1/4 cup fresh mint leaves
- 1/2 cup low-fat cottage cheese
- 1/3 cup water or breast milk/formula

Instructions:

1. Steam apples until soft, about 8-10 minutes.
2. Place steamed apples, mint leaves, cottage cheese, and water or breast milk/formula in a blender.
3. Puree until smooth, adding more liquid if needed.
4. Serve immediately or refrigerate.

Nutritional Information (per serving):
Calories: 90 | Carbohydrates: 18g | Protein: 4g | Fiber: 2g | Fat: 1.5g | Sodium: 150mg | Sugar: 14g | Calcium: 80mg | Iron: 0.3mg | Potassium: 140mg

Banana + Coconut Milk + Cinnamon Baby Food Puree

Prep Time: 5 minutes | **Cooking Time:** 0 minutes | **Per Serving:** 4 servings

Ingredients:

- 2 ripe bananas
- 1/2 cup coconut milk (full-fat)
- 1/2 teaspoon ground cinnamon

Instructions:

1. Place bananas, coconut milk, and cinnamon in a blender.
2. Puree until smooth and creamy.
3. Serve immediately or refrigerate.

Nutritional Information (per serving):
Calories: 120 | Carbohydrates: 27g | Protein: 1g | Fiber: 3g | Fat: 4g | Sodium: 10mg | Sugar: 14g | Calcium: 10mg | Iron: 0.3mg | Potassium: 350mg

Yogurt Nog Smoothie

Prep Time: 5 minutes | **Cooking Time:** 0 minutes | **Per Serving:** 1

Ingredients:

- 1 cup plain Greek yogurt
- 1/2 cup milk (dairy or plant-based)
- 1/2 teaspoon vanilla extract
- 1/4 teaspoon ground nutmeg
- 1/4 teaspoon ground cinnamon
- 1 tablespoon honey or maple syrup (optional)

Instructions:

1. Combine all ingredients in a blender.
2. Blend until smooth and creamy.
3. Taste and adjust sweetness if desired.
4. Serve immediately.

Nutritional Information (per serving):
Calories: 180 | Carbohydrates: 15g | Protein: 15g | Fiber: 0g | Fat: 4g | Sodium: 80mg | Sugar: 12g | Calcium: 250mg | Iron: 0.1mg | Potassium: 350mg

Hawaiian Shake

Prep Time: 5 minutes | **Cooking Time:** 0 minutes | **Per Serving:** 1

Ingredients:

- 1 cup pineapple chunks (fresh or frozen)
- 1/2 cup coconut milk
- 1/2 cup plain or vanilla yogurt
- 1 tablespoon honey (optional)
- 1/2 teaspoon vanilla extract
- Ice cubes (optional)

Instructions:

1. Combine pineapple, coconut milk, yogurt, honey, and vanilla extract in a blender.

2. Blend until smooth and creamy.
3. Add ice cubes if desired and blend again.
4. Serve immediately.

Nutritional Information (per serving):
Calories: 220 | Carbohydrates: 35g | Protein: 6g | Fiber: 2g | Fat: 5g | Sodium: 50mg | Sugar: 28g | Calcium: 200mg | Iron: 0.3mg | Potassium: 300mg

Honey Shake

Prep Time: 5 minutes | **Cooking Time:** 0 minutes | **Per Serving:** 1

Ingredients:

- 1 cup milk (dairy or plant-based)
- 2 tablespoons honey
- 1/2 teaspoon vanilla extract
- 1/2 cup plain yogurt
- Ice cubes (optional)

Instructions:

1. Add milk, honey, vanilla extract, and yogurt to a blender.
2. Blend until smooth.
3. Add ice cubes if desired and blend again.
4. Serve immediately.

Nutritional Information (per serving):
Calories: 210 | Carbohydrates: 30g | Protein: 8g | Fiber: 0g | Fat: 4g | Sodium: 100mg | Sugar: 28g | Calcium: 250mg | Iron: 0.1mg | Potassium: 350mg

Malted Milk Smoothie

Prep Time: 5 minutes | **Cooking Time:** 0 minutes | **Per Serving:** 1

Ingredients:

- 1 cup milk (dairy or plant-based)
- 2 tablespoons malted milk powder
- 1/2 cup vanilla ice cream or frozen yogurt
- 1/2 teaspoon vanilla extract
- Ice cubes (optional)

Instructions:

1. Combine milk, malted milk powder, ice cream, and vanilla extract in a blender.
2. Blend until smooth and creamy.
3. Add ice cubes if desired and blend again.
4. Serve immediately.

Nutritional Information (per serving):
Calories: 320 | Carbohydrates: 40g | Protein: 9g | Fiber: 0g | Fat: 10g | Sodium: 150mg | Sugar: 35g | Calcium: 300mg | Iron: 0.2mg | Potassium: 400mg

Nutty Chocolate Milkshake

Prep Time: 5 minutes | **Cooking Time:** 0 minutes | **Per Serving:** 1

Ingredients:

- 1 cup chocolate milk (dairy or plant-based)
- 2 tablespoons peanut butter or almond butter
- 1/2 cup vanilla ice cream or frozen yogurt
- 1 tablespoon cocoa powder
- Ice cubes (optional)

Instructions:

1. Add chocolate milk, nut butter, ice cream, and cocoa powder to a blender.
2. Blend until smooth and creamy.
3. Add ice cubes if desired and blend again.
4. Serve immediately.

Nutritional Information (per serving):
Calories: 400 | Carbohydrates: 45g | Protein: 12g | Fiber: 3g | Fat: 15g | Sodium: 150mg | Sugar: 38g | Calcium: 300mg | Iron: 1mg | Potassium: 450mg

Vanilla Milkshake

Prep Time: 5 minutes | **Cooking Time:** 0 minutes | **Per Serving:** 1

Ingredients:

- 1 cup milk (dairy or plant-based)
- 1/2 cup vanilla ice cream or frozen yogurt
- 1 teaspoon vanilla extract
- 1 tablespoon honey or sugar (optional)
- Ice cubes (optional)

Instructions:

1. Combine milk, ice cream, vanilla extract, and honey or sugar in a blender.
2. Blend until smooth and creamy.
3. Add ice cubes if desired and blend again.
4. Serve immediately.

Nutritional Information (per serving):
Calories: 280 | Carbohydrates: 35g | Protein: 8g | Fiber: 0g | Fat: 8g | Sodium: 120mg | Sugar: 30g | Calcium: 280mg | Iron: 0.1mg | Potassium: 350mg

Chapter 5

Lunch and Dinner

Creamy Roasted Cauliflower Soup

Prep Time: 10 minutes | **Cooking Time:** 40 minutes | **Per Serving:** 4

Ingredients:

- 1 large head cauliflower, cut into florets
- 2 tablespoons olive oil
- 1 medium onion, chopped
- 2 garlic cloves, minced
- 4 cups low-sodium vegetable broth
- 1 cup unsweetened almond milk or milk of choice
- 1/2 teaspoon ground nutmeg
- Salt and pepper, to taste
- Fresh chives or parsley, for garnish (optional)

Instructions:

1. Preheat oven to 425°F (220°C).
2. Toss cauliflower florets with 1 tablespoon olive oil, salt, and pepper. Spread on a baking sheet and roast for 25–30 minutes, until golden and tender.
3. In a large pot, heat remaining olive oil over medium heat. Add onion and garlic; sauté until soft, about 5 minutes.
4. Add roasted cauliflower and vegetable broth. Bring to a simmer and cook for 10 minutes.
5. Stir in almond milk and nutmeg. Remove from heat.
6. Puree soup using an immersion blender or in batches in a blender until smooth.
7. Season with salt and pepper to taste.
8. Serve hot, garnished with chives or parsley if desired.

Nutritional Information (per serving):
Calories: 130 | Carbohydrates: 18g | Protein: 5g | Fiber: 5g | Fat: 6g | Sodium: 350mg | Sugar: 5g | Calcium: 80mg | Iron: 1.2mg | Potassium: 600mg

SheetPan Tomato Soup

Prep Time: 10 minutes | **Cooking Time:** 35 minutes | **Per Serving:** 4

Ingredients:

- 2 pounds ripe tomatoes, halved
- 1 medium onion, quartered
- 4 garlic cloves, peeled
- 2 tablespoons olive oil
- 2 cups low-sodium vegetable broth
- 1 teaspoon dried basil
- 1 teaspoon dried oregano
- Salt and pepper, to taste
- 1/2 cup plain Greek yogurt or cream (optional, for creaminess)
- Fresh basil, for garnish (optional)

Instructions:

1. Preheat oven to 425°F (220°C).
2. Arrange tomatoes, onion, and garlic on a sheet pan. Drizzle with olive oil, salt, and pepper.
3. Roast for 25–30 minutes, until vegetables are soft and caramelized.
4. Transfer roasted vegetables to a blender. Add vegetable broth, basil, and oregano. Puree until smooth.
5. Pour into a pot, heat gently, and stir in Greek yogurt or cream if using.

6. Adjust seasoning as needed.
7. Serve hot, garnished with fresh basil.

Nutritional Information (per serving):
Calories: 110 | Carbohydrates: 18g | Protein: 4g | Fiber: 4g | Fat: 4g | Sodium: 320mg | Sugar: 10g | Calcium: 60mg | Iron: 1mg | Potassium: 700mg

Creamy Corn Soup with Jalapeños

Prep Time: 10 minutes | **Cooking Time:** 25 minutes | **Per Serving:** 4

Ingredients:

- 4 cups corn kernels (fresh or frozen)
- 1 medium onion, chopped
- 1 jalapeño, seeded and chopped
- 2 tablespoons butter or olive oil
- 3 cups low-sodium vegetable broth
- 1 cup milk or unsweetened plant-based milk
- 1/2 teaspoon ground cumin
- Salt and pepper, to taste
- Chopped cilantro, for garnish (optional)

Instructions:

1. In a large pot, melt butter over medium heat. Add onion and jalapeño; sauté until soft, about 5 minutes.
2. Add corn, cumin, salt, and pepper. Cook for 3 minutes.
3. Pour in vegetable broth and bring to a boil. Reduce heat and simmer for 10 minutes.
4. Stir in milk and remove from heat.
5. Puree soup using an immersion blender or in batches until smooth.
6. Adjust seasoning as needed.
7. Serve hot, garnished with cilantro if desired.

Nutritional Information (per serving):
Calories: 180 | Carbohydrates: 32g | Protein: 5g | Fiber: 4g | Fat: 6g | Sodium: 300mg | Sugar: 8g | Calcium: 70mg | Iron: 1mg | Potassium: 400mg

Easy Creamy Vegetable Soup

Prep Time: 10 minutes | **Cooking Time:** 25 minutes | **Per Serving:** 4

Ingredients:

- 2 cups broccoli florets
- 2 carrots, peeled and chopped
- 1 zucchini, chopped
- 1 medium potato, peeled and diced
- 1 small onion, chopped
- 2 tablespoons olive oil
- 4 cups low-sodium vegetable broth
- 1 cup milk or unsweetened plant-based milk
- Salt and pepper, to taste
- Fresh dill or parsley, for garnish (optional)

Instructions:

1. In a large pot, heat olive oil over medium heat. Add onion, carrots, broccoli, zucchini, and potato; sauté for 5 minutes.
2. Add vegetable broth and bring to a boil. Reduce heat and simmer for 15–20 minutes, until vegetables are tender.
3. Stir in milk and remove from heat.
4. Puree soup until smooth using an immersion blender or in batches.
5. Season with salt and pepper to taste.
6. Serve hot, garnished with dill or parsley if desired.

Nutritional Information (per serving):
Calories: 140 | Carbohydrates: 25g | Protein: 5g | Fiber: 5g | Fat: 4g | Sodium: 300mg | Sugar: 7g | Calcium: 80mg | Iron: 1.2mg | Potassium: 650mg

Velvety Butternut and Cauliflower Soup

Prep Time: 10 minutes | **Cooking Time:** 30 minutes | **Per Serving:** 4

Ingredients:

- 1 small butternut squash, peeled and cubed
- 1/2 head cauliflower, cut into florets
- 1 medium onion, chopped
- 2 tablespoons olive oil
- 4 cups low-sodium vegetable broth
- 1 cup coconut milk or milk of choice
- 1/2 teaspoon ground nutmeg
- Salt and pepper, to taste
- Pumpkin seeds, for garnish (optional)

Instructions:

1. In a large pot, heat olive oil over medium heat. Add onion; sauté until soft, about 5 minutes.
2. Add butternut squash and cauliflower; cook for 3 minutes.
3. Pour in vegetable broth, bring to a boil, then reduce heat and simmer for 20 minutes until vegetables are tender.
4. Stir in coconut milk and nutmeg. Remove from heat.
5. Puree soup until smooth.
6. Season with salt and pepper to taste.
7. Serve hot, garnished with pumpkin seeds if desired.

Nutritional Information (per serving):
Calories: 160 | Carbohydrates: 24g | Protein: 4g | Fiber: 5g | Fat: 6g | Sodium: 320mg | Sugar: 7g | Calcium: 70mg | Iron: 1.4mg | Potassium: 500mg

Moroccan Pureed Vegetable Soup

Prep Time: 10 minutes | **Cooking Time:** 30 minutes | **Per Serving:** 4

Ingredients:

- 2 carrots, peeled and chopped
- 1 sweet potato, peeled and diced
- 1 zucchini, chopped
- 1 small onion, chopped
- 2 tablespoons olive oil
- 1 teaspoon ground cumin
- 1/2 teaspoon ground coriander
- 1/2 teaspoon ground cinnamon
- 4 cups low-sodium vegetable broth
- Salt and pepper, to taste
- Fresh cilantro, for garnish (optional)

Instructions:

1. In a large pot, heat olive oil over medium heat. Add onion, carrots, sweet potato, and zucchini; sauté for 5 minutes.
2. Stir in cumin, coriander, and cinnamon; cook for 1 minute.
3. Add vegetable broth, bring to a boil, then reduce heat and simmer for 20–25 minutes until vegetables are soft.
4. Puree soup until smooth.
5. Season with salt and pepper to taste.
6. Serve hot, garnished with cilantro if desired.

Nutritional Information (per serving):
Calories: 130 | Carbohydrates: 27g | Protein: 3g | Fiber: 5g | Fat: 4g | Sodium: 320mg | Sugar: 9g | Calcium: 60mg | Iron: 1.1mg | Potassium: 450mg

Puree of Winter Vegetable Soup

Prep Time: 10 minutes | **Cooking Time:** 30 minutes | **Per Serving:** 4

Ingredients:

- 2 parsnips, peeled and chopped
- 2 carrots, peeled and chopped
- 1 small turnip, peeled and cubed
- 1 small potato, peeled and diced
- 1 small onion, chopped
- 2 tablespoons olive oil
- 4 cups low-sodium vegetable broth
- 1 cup milk or unsweetened plant-based milk
- Salt and pepper, to taste
- Chopped chives, for garnish (optional)

Instructions:

1. In a large pot, heat olive oil over medium heat. Add onion, parsnips, carrots, turnip, and potato; sauté for 5 minutes.
2. Add vegetable broth, bring to a boil, then reduce heat and simmer for 20–25 minutes until vegetables are very tender.
3. Stir in milk and remove from heat.
4. Puree soup until smooth.
5. Season with salt and pepper to taste.
6. Serve hot, garnished with chives if desired.

Nutritional Information (per serving):
Calories: 150 | Carbohydrates: 29g | Protein: 4g | Fiber: 6g | Fat: 4g | Sodium: 310mg | Sugar: 8g | Calcium: 70mg | Iron: 1mg | Potassium: 600mg

Broccoli and Spinach Pureed Soup

Prep Time: 10 minutes | **Cooking Time:** 20 minutes | **Per Serving:** 4

Ingredients:

- 1 tablespoon olive oil
- 1 medium onion, chopped
- 2 garlic cloves, minced
- 4 cups broccoli florets
- 2 cups fresh spinach leaves
- 4 cups low-sodium vegetable broth
- 1 cup milk or unsweetened plant-based milk
- Salt and pepper, to taste
- Lemon juice, to taste (optional)
- Fresh parsley, for garnish (optional)

Instructions:

1. In a large pot, heat olive oil over medium heat. Add onion and garlic; sauté until soft, about 5 minutes.
2. Add broccoli and vegetable broth. Bring to a boil, then reduce heat and simmer for 10 minutes, until broccoli is tender.
3. Add spinach and cook for 2 more minutes, until wilted.
4. Stir in milk and remove from heat.
5. Puree soup until smooth using an immersion blender or in batches.
6. Season with salt, pepper, and lemon juice to taste.
7. Serve hot, garnished with parsley if desired.

Nutritional Information (per serving):
Calories: 110 | Carbohydrates: 17g | Protein: 6g | Fiber: 4g | Fat: 3g | Sodium: 320mg | Sugar: 6g | Calcium: 110mg | Iron: 1.6mg | Potassium: 600mg

Carrot and Ginger Pureed Soup

Prep Time: 10 minutes | **Cooking Time:** 25 minutes | **Per Serving:** 4

Ingredients:

- 1 tablespoon olive oil
- 1 medium onion, chopped
- 1 tablespoon fresh ginger, grated
- 5 large carrots, peeled and sliced
- 4 cups low-sodium vegetable broth
- 1 cup orange juice
- Salt and pepper, to taste
- Fresh cilantro or parsley, for garnish (optional)

Instructions:

1. In a large pot, heat olive oil over medium heat. Add onion and ginger; sauté for 3 minutes.
2. Add carrots and cook for 2 minutes more.
3. Pour in vegetable broth and bring to a boil. Reduce heat and simmer for 15–20 minutes, until carrots are very tender.
4. Stir in orange juice and remove from heat.
5. Puree soup until smooth.
6. Season with salt and pepper to taste.
7. Serve hot, garnished with cilantro or parsley if desired.

Nutritional Information (per serving):
Calories: 120 | Carbohydrates: 26g | Protein: 2g | Fiber: 4g | Fat: 3g | Sodium: 300mg | Sugar: 14g | Calcium: 60mg | Iron: 0.5mg | Potassium: 600mg

Potato and Leek Pureed Soup

Prep Time: 10 minutes | **Cooking Time:** 30 minutes | **Per Serving:** 4

Ingredients:

- 2 tablespoons butter or olive oil
- 2 large leeks, white and light green parts only, sliced
- 3 medium potatoes, peeled and diced
- 4 cups low-sodium vegetable broth
- 1 cup milk or unsweetened plant-based milk
- Salt and pepper, to taste
- Chives, for garnish (optional)

Instructions:

1. In a large pot, melt butter over medium heat. Add leeks and cook until soft, about 5 minutes.
2. Add potatoes and broth. Bring to a boil, then reduce heat and simmer for 20 minutes, until potatoes are very tender.
3. Stir in milk and remove from heat.
4. Puree soup until smooth.
5. Season with salt and pepper to taste.
6. Serve hot, garnished with chives if desired.

Nutritional Information (per serving):
Calories: 170 | Carbohydrates: 32g | Protein: 4g | Fiber: 4g | Fat: 4g | Sodium: 320mg | Sugar: 5g | Calcium: 60mg | Iron: 1mg | Potassium: 750mg

Roasted Red Pepper and Tomato Puree

Prep Time: 10 minutes | **Cooking Time:** 30 minutes | **Per Serving:** 4

Ingredients:

- 3 red bell peppers, halved and seeded
- 4 large tomatoes, halved
- 1 medium onion, quartered
- 3 garlic cloves, peeled
- 2 tablespoons olive oil
- 2 cups low-sodium vegetable broth
- 1 teaspoon smoked paprika
- Salt and pepper, to taste
- Fresh basil, for garnish (optional)

Instructions:

1. Preheat oven to 425°F (220°C).
2. Arrange peppers, tomatoes, onion, and garlic on a baking sheet. Drizzle with olive oil and season with salt and pepper.
3. Roast for 25–30 minutes, until vegetables are soft and slightly charred.
4. Transfer vegetables to a blender. Add broth and smoked paprika. Puree until smooth.
5. Pour into a pot and heat gently if needed.
6. Serve hot, garnished with fresh basil if desired.

Nutritional Information (per serving):
Calories: 110 | Carbohydrates: 20g | Protein: 3g | Fiber: 5g | Fat: 4g | Sodium: 260mg | Sugar: 10g | Calcium: 40mg | Iron: 1mg | Potassium: 700mg

Sweet Potato and Apple Puree

Prep Time: 10 minutes | **Cooking Time:** 20 minutes | **Per Serving:** 4

Ingredients:

- 2 medium sweet potatoes, peeled and diced
- 2 apples, peeled, cored, and chopped
- 1/2 teaspoon ground cinnamon
- 2 cups water or low-sodium vegetable broth
- 1 tablespoon maple syrup (optional)

Instructions:

1. In a medium saucepan, combine sweet potatoes, apples, and water or broth.
2. Bring to a boil, then reduce heat and simmer for 15–20 minutes, until both are very tender.
3. Add cinnamon and maple syrup if using.
4. Puree mixture until smooth.
5. Serve warm or chilled.

Nutritional Information (per serving):
Calories: 110 | Carbohydrates: 26g | Protein: 1g | Fiber: 4g | Fat: 0g | Sodium: 30mg | Sugar: 11g | Calcium: 30mg | Iron: 0.4mg | Potassium: 350mg

Creamy Mushroom Soup Puree

Prep Time: 10 minutes | **Cooking Time:** 25 minutes | **Per Serving:** 4

Ingredients:

- 2 tablespoons butter or olive oil
- 1 medium onion, chopped
- 3 cups mushrooms, sliced
- 2 garlic cloves, minced
- 4 cups low-sodium vegetable broth
- 1 cup milk or unsweetened plant-based milk
- 1 teaspoon dried thyme
- Salt and pepper, to taste
- Fresh parsley, for garnish (optional)

Instructions:

1. In a large pot, melt butter over medium heat. Add onion and garlic; sauté until soft, about 5 minutes.
2. Add mushrooms and thyme; cook until mushrooms are browned, about 8 minutes.
3. Pour in broth and bring to a boil. Reduce heat and simmer for 10 minutes.
4. Stir in milk and remove from heat.
5. Puree soup until smooth.
6. Season with salt and pepper to taste.
7. Serve hot, garnished with parsley if desired.

Nutritional Information (per serving):
Calories: 120 | Carbohydrates: 14g | Protein: 5g | Fiber: 3g | Fat: 6g | Sodium: 300mg | Sugar: 6g | Calcium: 70mg | Iron: 1mg | Potassium: 500mg

Parsnip and Celery Root Puree

Prep Time: 10 minutes | **Cooking Time:** 20 minutes | **Per Serving:** 4

Ingredients:

- 2 large parsnips, peeled and chopped
- 1 small celery root (celeriac), peeled and chopped
- 2 tablespoons butter or olive oil
- 2 cups low-sodium vegetable broth
- 1/2 cup milk or unsweetened plant-based milk
- Salt and pepper, to taste
- Chopped chives or parsley, for garnish (optional)

Instructions:

1. In a medium saucepan, combine parsnips, celery root, and broth.
2. Bring to a boil, then reduce heat and simmer for 15–20 minutes, until vegetables are very tender.
3. Drain excess broth if needed, then add butter and milk.
4. Puree until smooth and creamy.
5. Season with salt and pepper to taste.
6. Serve warm, garnished with chives or parsley if desired.

Nutritional Information (per serving):
Calories: 130 | Carbohydrates: 23g | Protein: 2g | Fiber: 5g | Fat: 5g | Sodium: 180mg | Sugar: 7g | Calcium: 50mg | Iron: 0.6mg | Potassium: 500mg

Roasted Pumpkin and Sage Puree

Prep Time: 10 minutes | **Cooking Time:** 30 minutes | **Per Serving:** 4

Ingredients:

- 1 small pumpkin or 2 cups pumpkin cubes
- 2 tablespoons olive oil
- 1 tablespoon fresh sage leaves, chopped (or 1 teaspoon dried sage)
- 1/2 cup low-sodium vegetable broth or water
- Salt and pepper, to taste

Instructions:

1. Preheat oven to 400°F (200°C).
2. Toss pumpkin cubes with olive oil, sage, salt, and pepper.
3. Spread on a baking sheet and roast for 25-30 minutes until tender and caramelized.
4. Transfer roasted pumpkin to a blender, add broth or water, and puree until smooth.
5. Adjust seasoning and consistency with more broth if needed.
6. Serve warm.

Nutritional Information (per serving):
Calories: 110 | Carbohydrates: 22g | Protein: 2g | Fiber: 3g | Fat: 4g | Sodium: 150mg | Sugar: 5g | Calcium: 40mg | Iron: 0.7mg | Potassium: 400mg

Cauliflower and White Bean Puree

Prep Time: 10 minutes | **Cooking Time:** 25 minutes | **Per Serving:** 4

Ingredients:

- 1 head cauliflower, cut into florets
- 1 cup cooked white beans (cannellini or navy beans)
- 2 garlic cloves, minced
- 2 tablespoons olive oil
- 1/2 cup low-sodium vegetable broth
- Salt and pepper, to taste

Instructions:

1. Steam cauliflower until tender, about 10-15 minutes.
2. In a blender, combine steamed cauliflower, white beans, garlic, olive oil, and vegetable broth.
3. Puree until smooth and creamy.
4. Season with salt and pepper to taste.
5. Serve warm.

Nutritional Information (per serving):
Calories: 140 | Carbohydrates: 20g | Protein: 7g | Fiber: 7g | Fat: 6g | Sodium: 180mg | Sugar: 4g | Calcium: 60mg | Iron: 2mg | Potassium: 500mg

Pea and Mint Pureed Soup

Prep Time: 5 minutes | **Cooking Time:** 15 minutes | **Per Serving:** 4

Ingredients:

- 3 cups fresh or frozen peas
- 1 small onion, chopped
- 2 tablespoons olive oil
- 4 cups low-sodium vegetable broth
- 1/4 cup fresh mint leaves
- Salt and pepper, to taste
- Lemon juice, to taste (optional)

Instructions:

1. In a pot, heat olive oil over medium heat. Add onion and sauté until translucent, about 5 minutes.
2. Add peas and vegetable broth; bring to a boil. Reduce heat and simmer for 10 minutes.
3. Remove from heat, add mint leaves.
4. Puree soup until smooth.
5. Season with salt, pepper, and lemon juice as desired.
6. Serve warm.

Nutritional Information (per serving):
Calories: 110 | Carbohydrates: 20g | Protein: 7g | Fiber: 6g | Fat: 4g | Sodium: 300mg | Sugar: 6g | Calcium: 40mg | Iron: 2mg | Potassium: 350mg

Lentil and Carrot Puree

Prep Time: 10 minutes | **Cooking Time:** 25 minutes | **Per Serving:** 4

Ingredients:

- 1 cup red lentils, rinsed
- 3 large carrots, peeled and chopped
- 1 small onion, chopped
- 2 tablespoons olive oil
- 4 cups low-sodium vegetable broth
- 1/2 teaspoon ground cumin
- Salt and pepper, to taste

Instructions:

1. In a pot, heat olive oil over medium heat. Add onion and sauté until soft, about 5 minutes.
2. Add carrots, lentils, cumin, and vegetable broth. Bring to a boil.
3. Reduce heat and simmer for 20 minutes until lentils and carrots are tender.
4. Puree until smooth.
5. Season with salt and pepper to taste.
6. Serve warm.

Nutritional Information (per serving):
Calories: 180 | Carbohydrates: 30g | Protein: 12g | Fiber: 8g | Fat: 5g | Sodium: 320mg | Sugar: 7g | Calcium: 40mg | Iron: 3mg | Potassium: 500mg

Butternut Squash and Coconut Milk Puree

Prep Time: 10 minutes | **Cooking Time:** 30 minutes | **Per Serving:** 4

Ingredients:

- 1 medium butternut squash, peeled and cubed
- 1 cup coconut milk (full fat)
- 1 small onion, chopped
- 2 tablespoons olive oil
- 1/2 teaspoon ground ginger
- Salt and pepper, to taste

Instructions:

1. In a pot, heat olive oil over medium heat. Add onion and sauté until soft, about 5 minutes.
2. Add butternut squash and ground ginger; cook for 2 minutes.
3. Add enough water to cover squash and bring to a boil. Reduce heat and simmer until squash is tender, about 20 minutes.
4. Drain excess water, add coconut milk, and puree until smooth.
5. Season with salt and pepper to taste.
6. Serve warm.

Nutritional Information (per serving):
Calories: 160 | Carbohydrates: 25g | Protein: 3g | Fiber: 5g | Fat: 7g | Sodium: 100mg | Sugar: 5g | Calcium: 30mg | Iron: 1mg | Potassium: 450mg

Creamy Asparagus Puree

Prep Time: 10 minutes | **Cooking Time:** 15 minutes | **Per Serving:** 4

Ingredients:

- 1 bunch asparagus, trimmed and cut into pieces
- 1 small potato, peeled and diced
- 1 small onion, chopped
- 2 tablespoons butter or olive oil
- 3 cups low-sodium vegetable broth
- 1/2 cup milk or unsweetened plant-based milk
- Salt and pepper, to taste

Instructions:

1. In a pot, heat butter or olive oil over medium heat. Add onion and sauté until translucent, about 5 minutes.
2. Add asparagus, potato, and vegetable broth. Bring to a boil, then reduce heat and simmer until vegetables are tender, about 10 minutes.
3. Stir in milk and remove from heat.
4. Puree until smooth.
5. Season with salt and pepper to taste.
6. Serve warm.

Nutritional Information (per serving):
Calories: 110 | Carbohydrates: 18g | Protein: 4g | Fiber: 5g | Fat: 4g | Sodium: 280mg | Sugar: 5g | Calcium: 40mg | Iron: 1mg | Potassium: 450mg

Pureed Chicken and Vegetable Stew

Prep Time: 15 minutes | **Cooking Time:** 40 minutes | **Per Serving:** 4

Ingredients:

- 1 pound boneless, skinless chicken breast, diced
- 2 carrots, peeled and chopped
- 2 celery stalks, chopped
- 1 small onion, chopped
- 2 tablespoons olive oil
- 4 cups low-sodium chicken broth
- 1 cup peas (fresh or frozen)
- Salt and pepper, to taste

Instructions:

1. In a large pot, heat olive oil over medium heat. Add onion, carrots, and celery; sauté until softened, about 7 minutes.
2. Add chicken and cook until no longer pink, about 5 minutes.
3. Pour in chicken broth and bring to a boil. Reduce heat and simmer for 20 minutes.
4. Add peas and cook for 5 more minutes.
5. Puree stew until smooth, adding broth if needed to reach desired consistency.
6. Season with salt and pepper to taste.
7. Serve warm.

Nutritional Information (per serving):
Calories: 220 | Carbohydrates: 15g | Protein: 30g | Fiber: 4g | Fat: 5g | Sodium: 350mg | Sugar: 6g | Calcium: 40mg | Iron: 2mg | Potassium: 600mg

Pureed Beef and Root Vegetable Mash

Prep Time: 15 minutes | **Cooking Time:** 45 minutes | **Per Serving:** 4

Ingredients:

- 1 pound lean beef stew meat, cut into small pieces
- 2 large carrots, peeled and chopped
- 2 parsnips, peeled and chopped
- 2 medium potatoes, peeled and diced
- 1 small onion, chopped
- 2 tablespoons olive oil
- 2 cups low-sodium beef broth
- Salt and pepper, to taste

Instructions:

1. In a large pot, heat olive oil over medium heat. Add onion and cook until translucent, about 5 minutes.
2. Add beef and brown on all sides, about 8 minutes.
3. Add carrots, parsnips, potatoes, and beef broth. Bring to a boil, then reduce heat and simmer for 30 minutes or until beef and vegetables are tender.
4. Transfer mixture to a blender and puree until smooth, adding broth as needed for desired consistency.
5. Season with salt and pepper to taste.
6. Serve warm.

Nutritional Information (per serving):
Calories: 280 | Carbohydrates: 25g | Protein: 28g | Fiber: 5g | Fat: 8g | Sodium: 320mg | Sugar: 7g | Calcium: 50mg | Iron: 3mg | Potassium: 700mg

Pureed Turkey and Sweet Potato Casserole

Prep Time: 15 minutes | **Cooking Time:** 40 minutes | **Per Serving:** 4

Ingredients:

- 1 pound ground turkey
- 2 medium sweet potatoes, peeled and diced
- 1 small onion, chopped
- 1 cup low-sodium chicken broth
- 1/2 cup plain Greek yogurt
- 1 teaspoon dried thyme
- 2 tablespoons olive oil
- Salt and pepper, to taste

Instructions:

1. Preheat oven to 375°F (190°C).
2. In a skillet, heat olive oil over medium heat. Add onion and cook until translucent, about 5 minutes.
3. Add ground turkey and cook until browned, about 8 minutes. Season with salt, pepper, and thyme.
4. Boil sweet potatoes until tender, about 15 minutes. Drain.
5. Combine turkey mixture, sweet potatoes, chicken broth, and Greek yogurt in a large bowl.
6. Transfer to a baking dish and bake for 15 minutes.
7. Puree the casserole in a blender or food processor until smooth.
8. Serve warm.

Nutritional Information (per serving):
Calories: 320 | Carbohydrates: 28g | Protein: 30g | Fiber: 5g | Fat: 7g | Sodium: 350mg | Sugar: 6g | Calcium: 80mg | Iron: 3mg | Potassium: 650mg

Creamy Salmon and Potato Puree

Prep Time: 10 minutes | **Cooking Time:** 25 minutes | **Per Serving:** 4

Ingredients:

- 1 pound salmon fillet, skin removed
- 3 medium potatoes, peeled and diced
- 1/2 cup milk or unsweetened plant-based milk
- 2 tablespoons butter or olive oil
- 1 tablespoon fresh dill, chopped (optional)
- Salt and pepper, to taste

Instructions:

1. Steam or boil potatoes until tender, about 15 minutes.
2. Steam salmon until cooked through, about 10 minutes.
3. Combine potatoes, salmon, milk, and butter in a blender.
4. Puree until smooth and creamy.
5. Stir in dill if using.
6. Season with salt and pepper to taste.
7. Serve warm.

Nutritional Information (per serving):
Calories: 280 | Carbohydrates: 25g | Protein: 28g | Fiber: 3g | Fat: 9g | Sodium: 200mg | Sugar: 3g | Calcium: 40mg | Iron: 2mg | Potassium: 600mg

Pureed Lentil and Spinach Dahl

Prep Time: 10 minutes | **Cooking Time:** 30 minutes | **Per Serving:** 4

Ingredients:

- 1 cup red lentils, rinsed
- 2 cups fresh spinach leaves
- 1 small onion, chopped
- 2 garlic cloves, minced
- 1 tablespoon olive oil
- 1 teaspoon ground turmeric
- 1 teaspoon ground cumin
- 4 cups low-sodium vegetable broth
- Salt and pepper, to taste

Instructions:

1. In a pot, heat olive oil over medium heat. Add onion and garlic; sauté until soft, about 5 minutes.
2. Add turmeric and cumin; cook for 1 minute.
3. Add lentils and vegetable broth; bring to a boil.
4. Reduce heat and simmer for 20 minutes until lentils are soft.
5. Stir in spinach and cook until wilted, about 5 minutes.
6. Puree until smooth.
7. Season with salt and pepper to taste.
8. Serve warm.

Nutritional Information (per serving):
Calories: 190 | Carbohydrates: 30g | Protein: 14g | Fiber: 8g | Fat: 5g | Sodium: 320mg | Sugar: 4g | Calcium: 60mg | Iron: 4mg | Potassium: 600mg

Pureed Chickpea and Carrot Stew

Prep Time: 10 minutes | **Cooking Time:** 30 minutes | **Per Serving:** 4

Ingredients:

- 1 can (15 oz) chickpeas, drained and rinsed
- 3 large carrots, peeled and chopped
- 1 small onion, chopped
- 2 garlic cloves, minced
- 2 tablespoons olive oil
- 1 teaspoon ground cumin
- 4 cups low-sodium vegetable broth
- Salt and pepper, to taste

Instructions:

1. Heat olive oil in a pot over medium heat. Add onion and garlic; sauté until soft, about 5 minutes.
2. Add carrots, cumin, chickpeas, and vegetable broth. Bring to a boil.
3. Reduce heat and simmer for 20 minutes until carrots are tender.
4. Puree until smooth.
5. Season with salt and pepper to taste.
6. Serve warm.

Nutritional Information (per serving):
Calories: 180 | Carbohydrates: 30g | Protein: 8g | Fiber: 8g | Fat: 5g | Sodium: 320mg | Sugar: 7g | Calcium: 50mg | Iron: 3mg | Potassium: 500mg

Pureed Eggplant and Tomato Ragout

Prep Time: 10 minutes | **Cooking Time:** 30 minutes | **Per Serving:** 4

Ingredients:

- 1 medium eggplant, peeled and diced
- 4 large tomatoes, chopped
- 1 small onion, chopped
- 2 garlic cloves, minced
- 2 tablespoons olive oil
- 1 teaspoon dried oregano
- Salt and pepper, to taste
- Fresh basil, for garnish (optional)

Instructions:

1. Heat olive oil in a large pan over medium heat. Add onion and garlic; sauté until soft, about 5 minutes.
2. Add eggplant and cook for 10 minutes until softened.
3. Add tomatoes and oregano; simmer for 15 minutes until mixture thickens.
4. Transfer to a blender and puree until smooth.
5. Season with salt and pepper to taste.
6. Serve warm, garnished with fresh basil if desired.

Nutritional Information (per serving):
Calories: 120 | Carbohydrates: 20g | Protein: 3g | Fiber: 6g | Fat: 6g | Sodium: 200mg | Sugar: 10g | Calcium: 40mg | Iron: 1mg | Potassium: 500mg

Pureed Zucchini and Basil Soup

Prep Time: 10 minutes | **Cooking Time:** 20 minutes | **Per Serving:** 4

Ingredients:

- 3 medium zucchinis, chopped
- 1 small onion, chopped
- 2 garlic cloves, minced
- 2 tablespoons olive oil
- 4 cups low-sodium vegetable broth
- 1/4 cup fresh basil leaves
- Salt and pepper, to taste

Instructions:

1. Heat olive oil in a pot over medium heat. Add onion and garlic; sauté until soft, about 5 minutes.
2. Add zucchini and vegetable broth; bring to a boil.
3. Reduce heat and simmer for 15 minutes until zucchini is tender.
4. Add basil leaves and puree soup until smooth.
5. Season with salt and pepper to taste.
6. Serve warm.

Nutritional Information (per serving):
Calories: 90 | Carbohydrates: 15g | Protein: 3g | Fiber: 4g | Fat: 5g | Sodium: 280mg | Sugar: 7g | Calcium: 40mg | Iron: 1mg | Potassium: 450mg

Pureed Cauliflower and Cheese Bake

Prep Time: 15 minutes | **Cooking Time:** 35 minutes | **Per Serving:** 4

Ingredients:

- 1 head cauliflower, cut into florets
- 1 cup shredded cheddar cheese
- 1/2 cup milk or unsweetened plant-based milk
- 2 tablespoons butter
- 2 tablespoons all-purpose flour
- 1/2 teaspoon garlic powder
- Salt and pepper, to taste
- 1/4 cup breadcrumbs (optional, for topping)

Instructions:

1. Preheat oven to 375°F (190°C).
2. Steam cauliflower until tender, about 10-15 minutes.
3. In a saucepan, melt butter over medium heat. Stir in flour and cook for 1-2 minutes to make a roux.
4. Gradually whisk in milk, cooking until sauce thickens. Remove from heat and stir in cheese, garlic powder, salt, and pepper.
5. Puree steamed cauliflower until smooth, then mix with cheese sauce.
6. Pour mixture into a baking dish. Sprinkle breadcrumbs on top if using.
7. Bake for 20 minutes until bubbly and golden.
8. Serve warm.

Nutritional Information (per serving):
Calories: 250 | Carbohydrates: 15g | Protein: 12g | Fiber: 5g | Fat: 15g | Sodium: 400mg | Sugar: 5g | Calcium: 300mg | Iron: 1mg | Potassium: 500mg

Pureed Green Bean and Potato Medley

Prep Time: 10 minutes | **Cooking Time:** 25 minutes | **Per Serving:** 4

Ingredients:

- 2 cups green beans, trimmed
- 2 medium potatoes, peeled and diced
- 1 small onion, chopped
- 2 tablespoons olive oil
- 1/2 cup low-sodium vegetable broth
- Salt and pepper, to taste

Instructions:

1. Steam green beans and potatoes until tender, about 15-20 minutes.
2. In a pan, heat olive oil and sauté onion until soft, about 5 minutes.
3. Combine green beans, potatoes, and sautéed onion in a blender.
4. Add vegetable broth and puree until smooth.
5. Season with salt and pepper to taste.
6. Serve warm.

Nutritional Information (per serving):
Calories: 140 | Carbohydrates: 30g | Protein: 4g | Fiber: 6g | Fat: 5g | Sodium: 250mg | Sugar: 5g | Calcium: 40mg | Iron: 1mg | Potassium: 600mg

Pureed Carrot and Pea Side Dish

Prep Time: 10 minutes | **Cooking Time:** 20 minutes | **Per Serving:** 4

Ingredients:

- 3 large carrots, peeled and chopped
- 1 cup peas (fresh or frozen)
- 1 tablespoon butter or olive oil
- 1/4 cup water or low-sodium vegetable broth
- Salt and pepper, to taste

Instructions:

1. Steam carrots and peas until tender, about 15 minutes.
2. Transfer to a blender, add butter and water or broth.
3. Puree until smooth.
4. Season with salt and pepper to taste.
5. Serve warm.

Nutritional Information (per serving):
Calories: 90 | Carbohydrates: 18g | Protein: 4g | Fiber: 6g | Fat: 3g | Sodium: 150mg | Sugar: 7g | Calcium: 30mg | Iron: 1mg | Potassium: 350mg

Pureed Butternut Squash and Apple Mash

Prep Time: 10 minutes | **Cooking Time:** 25 minutes | **Per Serving:** 4

Ingredients:

- 2 cups butternut squash, peeled and cubed
- 2 apples, peeled, cored, and chopped
- 1/2 teaspoon ground cinnamon
- 1/4 cup water or low-sodium vegetable broth
- 1 tablespoon butter (optional)

Instructions:

1. Steam butternut squash and apples until tender, about 20 minutes.
2. Transfer to a blender, add cinnamon and water or broth.
3. Puree until smooth.
4. Stir in butter if using.
5. Serve warm.

Nutritional Information (per serving):
Calories: 110 | Carbohydrates: 28g | Protein: 1g | Fiber: 5g | Fat: 3g | Sodium: 30mg | Sugar: 15g | Calcium: 30mg | Iron: 0.4mg | Potassium: 400mg

Pureed Sweet Corn and Potato Chowder

Prep Time: 10 minutes | **Cooking Time:** 30 minutes | **Per Serving:** 4

Ingredients:

- 3 cups corn kernels (fresh or frozen)
- 2 medium potatoes, peeled and diced
- 1 small onion, chopped
- 2 tablespoons butter or olive oil
- 3 cups low-sodium vegetable broth
- 1 cup milk or unsweetened plant-based milk
- Salt and pepper, to taste

Instructions:

1. In a pot, heat butter or olive oil over medium heat. Add onion and sauté until soft, about 5 minutes.
2. Add corn, potatoes, and vegetable broth. Bring to a boil, then reduce heat and simmer until potatoes are tender, about 20 minutes.
3. Stir in milk and remove from heat.
4. Puree soup until smooth.
5. Season with salt and pepper to taste.
6. Serve warm.

Nutritional Information (per serving):
Calories: 180 | Carbohydrates: 35g | Protein: 5g | Fiber: 5g | Fat: 6g | Sodium: 320mg | Sugar: 8g | Calcium: 70mg | Iron: 1mg | Potassium: 500mg

Pureed Spinach and Potato Gratin

Prep Time: 15 minutes | **Cooking Time:** 40 minutes | **Per Serving:** 4

Ingredients:

- 3 cups fresh spinach leaves
- 3 medium potatoes, peeled and thinly sliced
- 1 cup shredded mozzarella or cheddar cheese
- 1 cup milk or unsweetened plant-based milk
- 2 tablespoons butter
- 2 cloves garlic, minced
- Salt and pepper, to taste

Instructions:

1. Preheat oven to 375°F (190°C).
2. Steam spinach until wilted, then chop finely.
3. In a saucepan, melt butter and sauté garlic until fragrant.
4. Layer potatoes and spinach in a baking dish, seasoning each layer with salt and pepper.
5. Pour milk over the layers and sprinkle cheese on top.
6. Cover with foil and bake for 30 minutes. Remove foil and bake another 10 minutes until cheese is golden.
7. Let cool slightly, then puree until smooth.
8. Serve warm.

Nutritional Information (per serving):
Calories: 250 | Carbohydrates: 30g | Protein: 15g | Fiber: 5g | Fat: 8g | Sodium: 400mg | Sugar: 4g | Calcium: 350mg | Iron: 3mg | Potassium: 700mg

Pureed Root Vegetable Medley

Prep Time: 10 minutes | **Cooking Time:** 30 minutes | **Per Serving:** 4

Ingredients:

- 2 carrots, peeled and chopped
- 2 parsnips, peeled and chopped
- 1 small turnip, peeled and chopped
- 1 small potato, peeled and diced
- 1 tablespoon olive oil
- 1/2 cup low-sodium vegetable broth
- Salt and pepper, to taste

Instructions:

1. Steam all vegetables until tender, about 20-25 minutes.
2. Transfer vegetables to a blender, add olive oil and vegetable broth.
3. Puree until smooth.
4. Season with salt and pepper to taste.
5. Serve warm.

Nutritional Information (per serving):
Calories: 140 | Carbohydrates: 30g | Protein: 3g | Fiber: 6g | Fat: 5g | Sodium: 150mg | Sugar: 8g | Calcium: 40mg | Iron: 1mg | Potassium: 600mg

Chapter 6

High Protein Pureed Meals

Pureed Chicken and Vegetable Medley

Prep Time: 15 minutes | **Cooking Time:** 35 minutes | **Per Serving:** 4

Ingredients:

- 1 pound boneless, skinless chicken breast, diced
- 2 carrots, peeled and chopped
- 1 cup green beans, trimmed and chopped
- 1 small onion, chopped
- 2 tablespoons olive oil
- 3 cups low-sodium chicken broth
- Salt and pepper, to taste

Instructions:

1. In a large pot, heat olive oil over medium heat. Add onion and sauté until translucent, about 5 minutes.
2. Add chicken and cook until no longer pink, about 7 minutes.
3. Add carrots, green beans, and chicken broth. Bring to a boil, then reduce heat and simmer for 20 minutes until vegetables are tender.
4. Transfer mixture to a blender and puree until smooth, adding broth as needed for desired consistency.
5. Season with salt and pepper to taste.
6. Serve warm.

Nutritional Information (per serving):
Calories: 220 | Carbohydrates: 15g | Protein: 30g | Fiber: 5g | Fat: 5g | Sodium: 350mg | Sugar: 6g | Calcium: 40mg | Iron: 2mg | Potassium: 600mg

Creamy Pureed Turkey and Sweet Potato

Prep Time: 15 minutes | **Cooking Time:** 40 minutes | **Per Serving:** 4

Ingredients:

- 1 pound ground turkey
- 2 medium sweet potatoes, peeled and diced
- 1 small onion, chopped
- 1 cup low-sodium chicken broth
- 1/2 cup plain Greek yogurt
- 1 teaspoon dried thyme
- 2 tablespoons olive oil
- Salt and pepper, to taste

Instructions:

1. In a skillet, heat olive oil over medium heat. Add onion and cook until translucent, about 5 minutes.
2. Add ground turkey and cook until browned, about 8 minutes. Season with salt, pepper, and thyme.
3. Boil sweet potatoes until tender, about 15 minutes. Drain.
4. Combine turkey mixture, sweet potatoes, chicken broth, and Greek yogurt in a blender.
5. Puree until smooth.
6. Serve warm.

Nutritional Information (per serving):
Calories: 320 | Carbohydrates: 28g | Protein: 30g | Fiber: 5g | Fat: 7g | Sodium: 350mg | Sugar: 6g | Calcium: 80mg | Iron: 3mg | Potassium: 650mg

Pureed Salmon and Cauliflower Mash

Prep Time: 10 minutes | **Cooking Time:** 25 minutes | **Per Serving:** 4

Ingredients:

- 1 pound salmon fillet, skin removed
- 1 head cauliflower, cut into florets
- 1/2 cup milk or unsweetened plant-based milk
- 2 tablespoons butter or olive oil
- 1 tablespoon fresh dill, chopped (optional)
- Salt and pepper, to taste

Instructions:

1. Steam or boil cauliflower until tender, about 10-15 minutes.
2. Steam salmon until cooked through, about 10 minutes.
3. Combine cauliflower, salmon, milk, and butter in a blender.
4. Puree until smooth and creamy.
5. Stir in dill if using.
6. Season with salt and pepper to taste.
7. Serve warm.

Nutritional Information (per serving):
Calories: 280 | Carbohydrates: 15g | Protein: 28g | Fiber: 5g | Fat: 9g | Sodium: 200mg | Sugar: 3g | Calcium: 40mg | Iron: 2mg | Potassium: 600mg

High-Protein Tofu and Spinach Puree

Prep Time: 10 minutes | **Cooking Time:** 10 minutes | **Per Serving:** 4

Ingredients:

- 1 block (14 oz) silken tofu
- 2 cups fresh spinach leaves
- 1 small onion, chopped
- 2 garlic cloves, minced
- 1 tablespoon olive oil
- 1/2 cup low-sodium vegetable broth
- Salt and pepper, to taste

Instructions:

1. In a pan, heat olive oil over medium heat. Add onion and garlic; sauté until soft, about 5 minutes.
2. Add spinach and cook until wilted, about 3 minutes.
3. Transfer spinach mixture, tofu, and vegetable broth to a blender.
4. Puree until smooth and creamy.
5. Season with salt and pepper to taste.
6. Serve warm.

Nutritional Information (per serving):
Calories: 180 | Carbohydrates: 8g | Protein: 15g | Fiber: 4g | Fat: 8g | Sodium: 200mg | Sugar: 2g | Calcium: 250mg | Iron: 3mg | Potassium: 400mg

Pureed Beef and Root Vegetable Stew

Prep Time: 15 minutes | **Cooking Time:** 45 minutes | **Per Serving:** 4

Ingredients:

- 1 pound lean beef stew meat, cut into small pieces
- 2 large carrots, peeled and chopped
- 2 parsnips, peeled and chopped
- 2 medium potatoes, peeled and diced
- 1 small onion, chopped
- 2 tablespoons olive oil
- 2 cups low-sodium beef broth
- Salt and pepper, to taste

Instructions:

1. Heat olive oil in a large pot over medium heat. Add onion and cook until translucent, about 5 minutes.
2. Add beef and brown on all sides, about 8 minutes.
3. Add carrots, parsnips, potatoes, and beef broth. Bring to a boil, then reduce heat and simmer for 30 minutes or until beef and vegetables are tender.
4. Puree stew until smooth, adding broth as needed for consistency.
5. Season with salt and pepper to taste.
6. Serve warm.

Nutritional Information (per serving):
Calories: 280 | Carbohydrates: 25g | Protein: 28g | Fiber: 5g | Fat: 8g | Sodium: 320mg | Sugar: 7g | Calcium: 50mg | Iron: 3mg | Potassium: 700mg

Pureed Lentil and Carrot Curry

Prep Time: 10 minutes | **Cooking Time:** 30 minutes | **Per Serving:** 4

Ingredients:

- 1 cup red lentils, rinsed
- 3 large carrots, peeled and chopped
- 1 small onion, chopped
- 2 tablespoons olive oil
- 1 teaspoon ground cumin
- 1 teaspoon ground turmeric
- 4 cups low-sodium vegetable broth
- Salt and pepper, to taste

Instructions:

1. Heat olive oil in a pot over medium heat. Add onion and sauté until soft, about 5 minutes.
2. Add cumin and turmeric; cook for 1 minute.
3. Add lentils, carrots, and vegetable broth. Bring to a boil.
4. Reduce heat and simmer for 20 minutes until lentils and carrots are tender.
5. Puree until smooth.
6. Season with salt and pepper to taste.
7. Serve warm.

Nutritional Information (per serving):
Calories: 180 | Carbohydrates: 30g | Protein: 12g | Fiber: 8g | Fat: 5g | Sodium: 320mg | Sugar: 7g | Calcium: 40mg | Iron: 3mg | Potassium: 500mg

Creamy Pureed Cottage Cheese and Peas

Prep Time: 5 minutes | **Cooking Time:** 15 minutes | **Per Serving:** 4

Ingredients:

- 1 cup low-fat cottage cheese
- 2 cups peas (fresh or frozen)
- 1/2 cup milk or unsweetened plant-based milk
- Salt and pepper, to taste

Instructions:

1. Steam peas until tender, about 10 minutes.
2. Combine peas, cottage cheese, and milk in a blender.
3. Puree until smooth and creamy.
4. Season with salt and pepper to taste.
5. Serve warm.

Nutritional Information (per serving):
Calories: 150 | Carbohydrates: 12g | Protein: 15g | Fiber: 5g | Fat: 4g | Sodium: 300mg | Sugar: 5g | Calcium: 200mg | Iron: 1mg | Potassium: 300mg

Pureed Egg and Cheese Casserole

Prep Time: 15 minutes | **Cooking Time:** 30 minutes | **Per Serving:** 4

Ingredients:

- 4 large eggs
- 1 cup shredded cheddar cheese
- 1/2 cup milk or unsweetened plant-based milk
- 1 small onion, finely chopped
- 1 tablespoon butter or olive oil
- Salt and pepper, to taste

Instructions:

1. Preheat oven to 350°F (175°C).
2. In a skillet, heat butter or olive oil and sauté onion until soft.
3. In a bowl, whisk eggs, milk, salt, and pepper. Stir in cheese and cooked onion.
4. Pour mixture into a greased baking dish.
5. Bake for 25-30 minutes until set.
6. Allow to cool slightly, then puree until smooth.
7. Serve warm.

Nutritional Information (per serving):
Calories: 250 | Carbohydrates: 5g | Protein: 20g | Fiber: 0g | Fat: 18g | Sodium: 400mg | Sugar: 2g | Calcium: 300mg | Iron: 2mg | Potassium: 250mg

Pureed White Fish and Potato Blend

Prep Time: 10 minutes | **Cooking Time:** 25 minutes | **Per Serving:** 4

Ingredients:

- 1 pound white fish fillets (cod, haddock), skin removed
- 3 medium potatoes, peeled and diced
- 1/2 cup milk or unsweetened plant-based milk
- 2 tablespoons butter or olive oil
- Salt and pepper, to taste

Instructions:

1. Steam or boil potatoes until tender, about 15 minutes.
2. Steam fish until cooked through, about 8-10 minutes.
3. Combine fish, potatoes, milk, and butter in a blender.
4. Puree until smooth and creamy.
5. Season with salt and pepper to taste.
6. Serve warm.

Nutritional Information (per serving):
Calories: 260 | Carbohydrates: 25g | Protein: 28g | Fiber: 3g | Fat: 7g | Sodium: 200mg | Sugar: 3g | Calcium: 40mg | Iron: 2mg | Potassium: 600mg

Pureed Black Bean and Quinoa Mash

Prep Time: 15 minutes | **Cooking Time:** 30 minutes | **Per Serving:** 4

Ingredients:

- 1 cup cooked black beans
- 1 cup cooked quinoa
- 1 small onion, chopped
- 2 garlic cloves, minced
- 2 tablespoons olive oil
- 1/2 cup low-sodium vegetable broth
- 1 teaspoon ground cumin
- Salt and pepper, to taste

Instructions:

1. Heat olive oil in a pan over medium heat. Add onion and garlic; sauté until soft, about 5 minutes.
2. In a blender, combine black beans, quinoa, sautéed onion and garlic, vegetable broth, and cumin.
3. Puree until smooth.
4. Season with salt and pepper to taste.
5. Serve warm.

Nutritional Information (per serving):
Calories: 280 | Carbohydrates: 40g | Protein: 15g | Fiber: 10g | Fat: 7g | Sodium: 250mg | Sugar: 3g | Calcium: 60mg | Iron: 4mg | Potassium: 600mg

Pureed Chicken Curry with Coconut Milk

Prep Time: 15 minutes | **Cooking Time:** 30 minutes | **Per Serving:** 4

Ingredients:

- 1 pound boneless, skinless chicken breast, diced
- 1 small onion, chopped
- 2 garlic cloves, minced
- 1 tablespoon olive oil
- 1 tablespoon curry powder
- 1 cup coconut milk (full fat)
- 2 cups low-sodium chicken broth
- Salt and pepper, to taste
- Fresh cilantro, for garnish (optional)

Instructions:

1. Heat olive oil in a pot over medium heat. Add onion and garlic; sauté until soft, about 5 minutes.
2. Add chicken and curry powder; cook until chicken is browned, about 8 minutes.
3. Pour in coconut milk and chicken broth. Bring to a boil, then reduce heat and simmer for 20 minutes until chicken is cooked through.
4. Puree soup until smooth.
5. Season with salt and pepper to taste.
6. Serve warm, garnished with cilantro if desired.

Nutritional Information (per serving):
Calories: 280 | Carbohydrates: 10g | Protein: 30g | Fiber: 3g | Fat: 15g | Sodium: 350mg | Sugar: 4g | Calcium: 40mg | Iron: 2mg | Potassium: 600mg

Pureed Turkey and Broccoli Bake

Prep Time: 15 minutes | **Cooking Time:** 40 minutes | **Per Serving:** 4

Ingredients:

- 1 pound ground turkey
- 2 cups broccoli florets
- 1 small onion, chopped
- 1/2 cup shredded cheddar cheese
- 1/2 cup low-sodium chicken broth
- 1/2 cup plain Greek yogurt
- 2 tablespoons olive oil
- Salt and pepper, to taste

Instructions:

1. Preheat oven to 375°F (190°C).
2. Heat olive oil in a skillet over medium heat. Add onion and cook until translucent, about 5 minutes.
3. Add ground turkey and cook until browned, about 8 minutes. Season with salt and pepper.
4. Steam broccoli until tender, about 5-7 minutes.
5. In a bowl, combine turkey mixture, broccoli, chicken broth, and Greek yogurt. Mix well.
6. Transfer to a baking dish, sprinkle cheese on top, and bake for 20 minutes until cheese is melted and bubbly.
7. Puree the casserole until smooth if needed.
8. Serve warm.

Nutritional Information (per serving):
Calories: 320 | Carbohydrates: 15g | Protein: 35g | Fiber: 5g | Fat: 10g | Sodium: 350mg | Sugar: 5g | Calcium: 250mg | Iron: 3mg | Potassium: 700mg

Pureed Creamy Ricotta and Zucchini

Prep Time: 10 minutes | **Cooking Time:** 15 minutes | **Per Serving:** 4

Ingredients:

- 2 medium zucchinis, chopped
- 1 cup ricotta cheese
- 1 small onion, chopped
- 1 tablespoon olive oil
- 1/2 cup low-sodium vegetable broth
- Salt and pepper, to taste
- Fresh basil, for garnish (optional)

Instructions:

1. Heat olive oil in a pan over medium heat. Add onion and sauté until soft, about 5 minutes.
2. Add zucchini and cook for 7-10 minutes until tender.
3. Transfer zucchini mixture, ricotta, and vegetable broth to a blender.
4. Puree until smooth and creamy.
5. Season with salt and pepper to taste.
6. Serve warm, garnished with basil if desired.

Nutritional Information (per serving):
Calories: 180 | Carbohydrates: 10g | Protein: 12g | Fiber: 3g | Fat: 10g | Sodium: 250mg | Sugar: 6g | Calcium: 300mg | Iron: 1mg | Potassium: 400mg

Pureed Tuna and Sweet Corn Chowder

Prep Time: 10 minutes | **Cooking Time:** 25 minutes | **Per Serving:** 4

Ingredients:

- 1 can (5 oz) tuna in water, drained
- 2 cups corn kernels (fresh or frozen)
- 2 medium potatoes, peeled and diced
- 1 small onion, chopped
- 2 tablespoons butter or olive oil
- 3 cups low-sodium vegetable broth
- 1 cup milk or unsweetened plant-based milk
- Salt and pepper, to taste

Instructions:

1. In a pot, heat butter or olive oil over medium heat. Add onion and sauté until soft, about 5 minutes.
2. Add corn, potatoes, and vegetable broth. Bring to a boil, then reduce heat and simmer until potatoes are tender, about 20 minutes.
3. Stir in milk and tuna.
4. Puree until smooth.
5. Season with salt and pepper to taste.
6. Serve warm.

Nutritional Information (per serving):
Calories: 250 | Carbohydrates: 30g | Protein: 25g | Fiber: 5g | Fat: 7g | Sodium: 350mg | Sugar: 6g | Calcium: 70mg | Iron: 2mg | Potassium: 600mg

Pureed Shrimp and Pumpkin Soup

Prep Time: 15 minutes | **Cooking Time:** 30 minutes | **Per Serving:** 4

Ingredients:

- 1 pound shrimp, peeled and deveined
- 2 cups pumpkin, peeled and cubed
- 1 small onion, chopped
- 2 garlic cloves, minced
- 2 tablespoons olive oil
- 4 cups low-sodium vegetable broth
- 1/2 cup coconut milk (optional)
- Salt and pepper, to taste

Instructions:

1. Heat olive oil in a pot over medium heat. Add onion and garlic; sauté until soft, about 5 minutes.
2. Add pumpkin and vegetable broth; bring to a boil. Reduce heat and simmer for 20 minutes until pumpkin is tender.
3. Add shrimp and cook until pink and opaque, about 5 minutes.
4. Remove from heat and puree soup until smooth.
5. Stir in coconut milk if using.
6. Season with salt and pepper to taste.
7. Serve warm.

Nutritional Information (per serving):
Calories: 220 | Carbohydrates: 18g | Protein: 28g | Fiber: 4g | Fat: 7g | Sodium: 320mg | Sugar: 6g | Calcium: 40mg | Iron: 2mg | Potassium: 550mg

Pureed Chickpea and Carrot Stew

Prep Time: 10 minutes | **Cooking Time:** 30 minutes | **Per Serving:** 4

Ingredients:

- 1 can (15 oz) chickpeas, drained and rinsed
- 3 large carrots, peeled and chopped
- 1 small onion, chopped
- 2 garlic cloves, minced
- 2 tablespoons olive oil
- 1 teaspoon ground cumin
- 4 cups low-sodium vegetable broth
- Salt and pepper, to taste

Instructions:

1. Heat olive oil in a pot over medium heat. Add onion and garlic; sauté until soft, about 5 minutes.
2. Add carrots, cumin, chickpeas, and vegetable broth. Bring to a boil.
3. Reduce heat and simmer for 20 minutes until carrots are tender.
4. Puree until smooth.
5. Season with salt and pepper to taste.
6. Serve warm.

Nutritional Information (per serving):
Calories: 180 | Carbohydrates: 30g | Protein: 8g | Fiber: 8g | Fat: 5g | Sodium: 320mg | Sugar: 7g | Calcium: 50mg | Iron: 3mg | Potassium: 500mg

Pureed Beef and Barley Soup

Prep Time: 15 minutes | **Cooking Time:** 45 minutes | **Per Serving:** 4

Ingredients:

- 1 pound lean beef stew meat, cut into small pieces
- 1/2 cup pearl barley
- 2 carrots, peeled and chopped
- 1 small onion, chopped
- 2 celery stalks, chopped
- 4 cups low-sodium beef broth
- 2 tablespoons olive oil
- Salt and pepper, to taste

Instructions:

1. Heat olive oil in a large pot over medium heat. Add onion and celery; sauté until soft, about 5 minutes.
2. Add beef and brown on all sides, about 8 minutes.
3. Add carrots, barley, and beef broth. Bring to a boil, then reduce heat and simmer for 30-40 minutes until beef and barley are tender.
4. Puree soup until smooth, adding broth if needed for desired consistency.
5. Season with salt and pepper to taste.
6. Serve warm.

Nutritional Information (per serving):
Calories: 300 | Carbohydrates: 30g | Protein: 28g | Fiber: 6g | Fat: 8g | Sodium: 350mg | Sugar: 6g | Calcium: 50mg | Iron: 4mg | Potassium: 700mg

Pureed Eggplant and Lentil Ragout

Prep Time: 10 minutes | **Cooking Time:** 35 minutes | **Per Serving:** 4

Ingredients:

- 1 medium eggplant, peeled and diced
- 1 cup red lentils, rinsed
- 1 small onion, chopped
- 2 garlic cloves, minced
- 2 tablespoons olive oil
- 1 teaspoon ground cumin
- 4 cups low-sodium vegetable broth
- Salt and pepper, to taste

Instructions:

1. Heat olive oil in a pot over medium heat. Add onion and garlic; sauté until soft, about 5 minutes.
2. Add eggplant and cook for 10 minutes until softened.
3. Add lentils, cumin, and vegetable broth. Bring to a boil.
4. Reduce heat and simmer for 20 minutes until lentils are tender.
5. Puree until smooth.
6. Season with salt and pepper to taste.
7. Serve warm.

Nutritional Information (per serving):
Calories: 220 | Carbohydrates: 35g | Protein: 14g | Fiber: 9g | Fat: 6g | Sodium: 320mg | Sugar: 7g | Calcium: 50mg | Iron: 4mg | Potassium: 600mg

Pureed Greek Yogurt and Cucumber Dip

Prep Time: 5 minutes | **Cooking Time:** 0 minutes | **Per Serving:** 4

Ingredients:

- 1 cup plain Greek yogurt
- 1 medium cucumber, peeled and chopped
- 1 garlic clove, minced
- 1 tablespoon fresh dill, chopped
- 1 tablespoon lemon juice
- Salt and pepper, to taste

Instructions:

1. Combine all ingredients in a blender.
2. Puree until smooth.
3. Season with salt and pepper to taste.
4. Chill before serving.
5. Serve as a dip or side dish.

Nutritional Information (per serving):
Calories: 80 | Carbohydrates: 5g | Protein: 8g | Fiber: 1g | Fat: 3g | Sodium: 60mg | Sugar: 4g | Calcium: 150mg | Iron: 0.3mg | Potassium: 150mg

Pureed Ham and Cheese Soup

Prep Time: 10 minutes | **Cooking Time:** 30 minutes | **Per Serving:** 4

Ingredients:

- 1 cup cooked ham, diced
- 1 small onion, chopped
- 2 cups potatoes, peeled and diced
- 2 cups low-sodium chicken broth
- 1 cup milk or unsweetened plant-based milk
- 1/2 cup shredded cheddar cheese
- 2 tablespoons butter or olive oil
- Salt and pepper, to taste

Instructions:

1. Heat butter or olive oil in a pot over medium heat. Add onion and sauté until soft, about 5 minutes.
2. Add ham, potatoes, and chicken broth. Bring to a boil, then reduce heat and simmer until potatoes are tender, about 20 minutes.
3. Stir in milk and cheese until melted.
4. Puree soup until smooth.
5. Season with salt and pepper to taste.
6. Serve warm.

Nutritional Information (per serving):
Calories: 300 | Carbohydrates: 25g | Protein: 25g | Fiber: 3g | Fat: 12g | Sodium: 600mg | Sugar: 5g | Calcium: 300mg | Iron: 2mg | Potassium: 600mg

Chapter 7

Vegetarian and Vegan Pureed Recipes

Creamy Sweet Potato and Coconut Puree

Prep Time: 10 minutes | **Cooking Time:** 25 minutes | **Per Serving:** 4

Ingredients:

- 2 medium sweet potatoes, peeled and diced
- 1 cup coconut milk (full fat)
- 1/2 teaspoon ground cinnamon
- 1 tablespoon maple syrup (optional)
- Pinch of salt

Instructions:

1. Steam or boil sweet potatoes until tender, about 20-25 minutes.
2. Transfer sweet potatoes to a blender. Add coconut milk, cinnamon, maple syrup (if using), and salt.
3. Puree until smooth and creamy.
4. Serve warm.

Nutritional Information (per serving):
Calories: 150 | Carbohydrates: 30g | Protein: 2g | Fiber: 4g | Fat: 6g | Sodium: 50mg | Sugar: 8g | Calcium: 40mg | Iron: 1mg | Potassium: 450mg

Roasted Cauliflower and Garlic Puree

Prep Time: 10 minutes | **Cooking Time:** 30 minutes | **Per Serving:** 4

Ingredients:

- 1 large head cauliflower, cut into florets
- 4 garlic cloves, peeled
- 2 tablespoons olive oil
- 1/2 cup low-sodium vegetable broth
- Salt and pepper, to taste

Instructions:

1. Preheat oven to 425°F (220°C).
2. Toss cauliflower and garlic with olive oil, salt, and pepper. Spread on a baking sheet and roast for 25-30 minutes until tender and golden.
3. Transfer roasted cauliflower and garlic to a blender. Add vegetable broth and puree until smooth.
4. Adjust seasoning and consistency as needed.
5. Serve warm.

Nutritional Information (per serving):
Calories: 120 | Carbohydrates: 15g | Protein: 5g | Fiber: 6g | Fat: 7g | Sodium: 200mg | Sugar: 5g | Calcium: 60mg | Iron: 1.2mg | Potassium: 500mg

Butternut Squash and Sage Puree

Prep Time: 10 minutes | **Cooking Time:** 30 minutes | **Per Serving:** 4

Ingredients:

- 1 medium butternut squash, peeled and cubed
- 1 tablespoon fresh sage, chopped (or 1 teaspoon dried sage)
- 2 tablespoons olive oil
- 1/2 cup low-sodium vegetable broth
- Salt and pepper, to taste

Instructions:

1. Preheat oven to 400°F (200°C).
2. Toss butternut squash with olive oil, sage, salt, and pepper. Spread on a baking sheet and roast for 25-30 minutes until tender.
3. Transfer to a blender, add vegetable broth, and puree until smooth.
4. Adjust seasoning and consistency as needed.
5. Serve warm.

Nutritional Information (per serving):
Calories: 140 | Carbohydrates: 28g | Protein: 2g | Fiber: 5g | Fat: 6g | Sodium: 150mg | Sugar: 7g | Calcium: 40mg | Iron: 0.8mg | Potassium: 450mg

Green Pea and Mint Puree

Prep Time: 5 minutes | **Cooking Time:** 15 minutes | **Per Serving:** 4

Ingredients:

- 3 cups fresh or frozen peas
- 1/4 cup fresh mint leaves
- 1/2 cup low-sodium vegetable broth
- 1 tablespoon olive oil
- Salt and pepper, to taste

Instructions:

1. Steam peas until tender, about 10 minutes.
2. Transfer peas, mint, vegetable broth, and olive oil to a blender.
3. Puree until smooth.
4. Season with salt and pepper to taste.
5. Serve warm.

Nutritional Information (per serving):
Calories: 110 | Carbohydrates: 20g | Protein: 7g | Fiber: 6g | Fat: 4g | Sodium: 200mg | Sugar: 6g | Calcium: 40mg | Iron: 2mg | Potassium: 350mg

Carrot and Ginger Puree

Prep Time: 10 minutes | **Cooking Time:** 25 minutes | **Per Serving:** 4

Ingredients:

- 5 large carrots, peeled and chopped
- 1 tablespoon fresh ginger, grated
- 1/2 cup low-sodium vegetable broth
- 1 tablespoon olive oil
- Salt and pepper, to taste

Instructions:

1. Steam carrots until tender, about 20 minutes.
2. Transfer carrots, ginger, vegetable broth, and olive oil to a blender.
3. Puree until smooth.
4. Season with salt and pepper to taste.
5. Serve warm.

Nutritional Information (per serving):
Calories: 120 | Carbohydrates: 26g | Protein: 2g | Fiber: 5g | Fat: 4g | Sodium: 150mg | Sugar: 12g | Calcium: 50mg | Iron: 0.5mg | Potassium: 600mg

Spinach and Avocado Puree

Prep Time: 5 minutes | **Cooking Time:** 5 minutes | **Per Serving:** 4

Ingredients:

- 2 cups fresh spinach leaves
- 1 ripe avocado
- 1/4 cup water or breast milk/formula
- 1 tablespoon lemon juice
- Salt and pepper, to taste (optional)

Instructions:

1. Steam spinach until wilted, about 3-5 minutes.
2. Transfer spinach, avocado, water or breast milk/formula, and lemon juice to a blender.
3. Puree until smooth and creamy.
4. Season with salt and pepper if desired.
5. Serve immediately.

Nutritional Information (per serving):
Calories: 140 | Carbohydrates: 8g | Protein: 3g | Fiber: 7g | Fat: 11g | Sodium: 50mg | Sugar: 1g | Calcium: 40mg | Iron: 1.5mg | Potassium: 500mg

Parsnip and Apple Puree

Prep Time: 10 minutes | **Cooking Time:** 20 minutes | **Per Serving:** 4

Ingredients:

- 3 large parsnips, peeled and chopped
- 2 apples, peeled, cored, and chopped
- 1/2 teaspoon ground cinnamon
- 1/4 cup water or low-sodium vegetable broth
- 1 tablespoon butter (optional)

Instructions:

1. Steam parsnips and apples until tender, about 20 minutes.
2. Transfer to a blender, add cinnamon and water or broth.
3. Puree until smooth.
4. Stir in butter if using.
5. Serve warm.

Nutritional Information (per serving):
Calories: 110 | Carbohydrates: 28g | Protein: 2g | Fiber: 5g | Fat: 3g | Sodium: 30mg | Sugar: 15g | Calcium: 30mg | Iron: 0.6mg | Potassium: 400mg

Zucchini and Basil Puree

Prep Time: 10 minutes | **Cooking Time:** 15 minutes | **Per Serving:** 4

Ingredients:

- 3 medium zucchinis, chopped
- 1/4 cup fresh basil leaves
- 1/2 cup low-sodium vegetable broth
- 1 tablespoon olive oil
- Salt and pepper, to taste

Instructions:

1. Steam zucchini until tender, about 10-12 minutes.
2. Transfer zucchini, basil, vegetable broth, and olive oil to a blender.
3. Puree until smooth.
4. Season with salt and pepper to taste.
5. Serve warm.

Nutritional Information (per serving):
Calories: 90 | Carbohydrates: 15g | Protein: 3g | Fiber: 4g | Fat: 5g | Sodium: 150mg | Sugar: 7g | Calcium: 40mg | Iron: 1mg | Potassium: 450mg

Broccoli and Cauliflower Mash

Prep Time: 10 minutes | **Cooking Time:** 20 minutes | **Per Serving:** 4

Ingredients:

- 2 cups broccoli florets
- 2 cups cauliflower florets
- 2 tablespoons butter or olive oil
- 1/4 cup low-sodium vegetable broth
- Salt and pepper, to taste

Instructions:

1. Steam broccoli and cauliflower until tender, about 15-20 minutes.
2. Transfer to a blender, add butter and vegetable broth.
3. Puree until smooth.
4. Season with salt and pepper to taste.
5. Serve warm.

Nutritional Information (per serving):
Calories: 110 | Carbohydrates: 15g | Protein: 6g | Fiber: 6g | Fat: 6g | Sodium: 150mg | Sugar: 5g | Calcium: 60mg | Iron: 1.5mg | Potassium: 500mg

Pumpkin and Cinnamon Puree

Prep Time: 10 minutes | **Cooking Time:** 25 minutes | **Per Serving:** 4

Ingredients:

- 2 cups pumpkin, peeled and cubed
- 1/2 teaspoon ground cinnamon
- 1/4 cup water or low-sodium vegetable broth
- 1 tablespoon maple syrup (optional)
- Pinch of salt

Instructions:

1. Steam pumpkin until tender, about 20-25 minutes.
2. Transfer pumpkin to a blender, add cinnamon, water or broth, maple syrup (if using), and salt.
3. Puree until smooth and creamy.
4. Serve warm.

Nutritional Information (per serving):
Calories: 110 | Carbohydrates: 26g | Protein: 2g | Fiber: 5g | Fat: 0g | Sodium: 50mg | Sugar: 8g | Calcium: 40mg | Iron: 1mg | Potassium: 400mg

Beetroot and Sweet Potato Puree

Prep Time: 10 minutes | **Cooking Time:** 30 minutes | **Per Serving:** 4

Ingredients:

- 2 medium beetroots, peeled and chopped
- 2 medium sweet potatoes, peeled and diced
- 1/4 cup water or low-sodium vegetable broth
- 1 tablespoon olive oil
- Salt and pepper, to taste

Instructions:

1. Steam beetroots and sweet potatoes until tender, about 25-30 minutes.
2. Transfer to a blender, add water or broth and olive oil.
3. Puree until smooth.
4. Season with salt and pepper to taste.
5. Serve warm.

Nutritional Information (per serving):
Calories: 140 | Carbohydrates: 32g | Protein: 3g | Fiber: 6g | Fat: 5g | Sodium: 50mg | Sugar: 10g | Calcium: 40mg | Iron: 1.2mg | Potassium: 600mg

Cauliflower and White Bean Puree

Prep Time: 10 minutes | **Cooking Time:** 25 minutes | **Per Serving:** 4

Ingredients:

- 1 head cauliflower, cut into florets
- 1 cup cooked white beans (cannellini or navy beans)
- 2 garlic cloves, minced
- 2 tablespoons olive oil
- 1/2 cup low-sodium vegetable broth
- Salt and pepper, to taste

Instructions:

1. Steam cauliflower until tender, about 10-15 minutes.
2. In a blender, combine steamed cauliflower, white beans, garlic, olive oil, and vegetable broth.
3. Puree until smooth and creamy.
4. Season with salt and pepper to taste.
5. Serve warm.

Nutritional Information (per serving):
Calories: 140 | Carbohydrates: 20g | Protein: 7g | Fiber: 7g | Fat: 6g | Sodium: 180mg | Sugar: 4g | Calcium: 60mg | Iron: 2mg | Potassium: 500mg

Kale and Potato Puree

Prep Time: 10 minutes | **Cooking Time:** 25 minutes | **Per Serving:** 4

Ingredients:

- 2 cups kale leaves, stems removed and chopped
- 3 medium potatoes, peeled and diced
- 2 tablespoons olive oil
- 1/2 cup low-sodium vegetable broth
- Salt and pepper, to taste

Instructions:

1. Steam kale and potatoes until tender, about 20-25 minutes.
2. Transfer to a blender, add olive oil and vegetable broth.
3. Puree until smooth.
4. Season with salt and pepper to taste.
5. Serve warm.

Nutritional Information (per serving):
Calories: 150 | Carbohydrates: 30g | Protein: 5g | Fiber: 6g | Fat: 7g | Sodium: 150mg | Sugar: 5g | Calcium: 80mg | Iron: 2mg | Potassium: 600mg

Lentil and Carrot Puree

Prep Time: 10 minutes | **Cooking Time:** 25 minutes | **Per Serving:** 4

Ingredients:

- 1 cup red lentils, rinsed
- 3 large carrots, peeled and chopped
- 1 small onion, chopped
- 2 tablespoons olive oil
- 4 cups low-sodium vegetable broth
- 1/2 teaspoon ground cumin
- Salt and pepper, to taste

Instructions:

1. Heat olive oil in a pot over medium heat. Add onion and sauté until soft, about 5 minutes.
2. Add carrots, lentils, cumin, and vegetable broth. Bring to a boil.
3. Reduce heat and simmer for 20 minutes until lentils and carrots are tender.
4. Puree until smooth.
5. Season with salt and pepper to taste.
6. Serve warm.

Nutritional Information (per serving):
Calories: 180 | Carbohydrates: 30g | Protein: 12g | Fiber: 8g | Fat: 5g | Sodium: 320mg | Sugar: 7g | Calcium: 40mg | Iron: 3mg | Potassium: 500mg

Sweet Corn and Potato Puree

Prep Time: 10 minutes | **Cooking Time:** 25 minutes | **Per Serving:** 4

Ingredients:

- 3 cups corn kernels (fresh or frozen)
- 2 medium potatoes, peeled and diced
- 1 small onion, chopped
- 2 tablespoons butter or olive oil
- 1/2 cup low-sodium vegetable broth
- Salt and pepper, to taste

Instructions:

1. Steam corn and potatoes until tender, about 20-25 minutes.
2. In a pan, heat butter or olive oil and sauté onion until soft, about 5 minutes.
3. Combine corn, potatoes, sautéed onion, and vegetable broth in a blender.
4. Puree until smooth.
5. Season with salt and pepper to taste.
6. Serve warm.

Nutritional Information (per serving):
Calories: 160 | Carbohydrates: 35g | Protein: 5g | Fiber: 5g | Fat: 6g | Sodium: 250mg | Sugar: 8g | Calcium: 50mg | Iron: 1mg | Potassium: 500mg

Roasted Red Pepper and Tomato Puree

Prep Time: 10 minutes | **Cooking Time:** 30 minutes | **Per Serving:** 4

Ingredients:

- 3 red bell peppers, halved and seeded
- 4 large tomatoes, halved
- 1 medium onion, quartered
- 3 garlic cloves, peeled
- 2 tablespoons olive oil
- 2 cups low-sodium vegetable broth
- 1 teaspoon smoked paprika
- Salt and pepper, to taste
- Fresh basil, for garnish (optional)

Instructions:

1. Preheat oven to 425°F (220°C).
2. Arrange peppers, tomatoes, onion, and garlic on a baking sheet. Drizzle with olive oil and season with salt and pepper.
3. Roast for 25-30 minutes until vegetables are soft and slightly charred.
4. Transfer to a blender, add broth and smoked paprika, and puree until smooth.
5. Heat gently if needed.
6. Serve warm, garnished with fresh basil if desired.

Nutritional Information (per serving):
Calories: 110 | Carbohydrates: 20g | Protein: 3g | Fiber: 5g | Fat: 4g | Sodium: 260mg | Sugar: 10g | Calcium: 40mg | Iron: 1mg | Potassium: 700mg

Butternut Squash and Coconut Milk Puree

Prep Time: 10 minutes | **Cooking Time:** 30 minutes | **Per Serving:** 4

Ingredients:

- 1 medium butternut squash, peeled and cubed
- 1 cup coconut milk (full fat)
- 1 small onion, chopped
- 2 tablespoons olive oil
- 1/2 teaspoon ground ginger
- Salt and pepper, to taste

Instructions:

1. Heat olive oil in a pot over medium heat. Add onion and sauté until soft, about 5 minutes.
2. Add butternut squash and ground ginger; cook for 2 minutes.
3. Add enough water to cover squash and bring to a boil. Reduce heat and simmer until squash is tender, about 20 minutes.
4. Drain excess water, add coconut milk, and puree until smooth.
5. Season with salt and pepper to taste.
6. Serve warm.

Nutritional Information (per serving):
Calories: 160 | Carbohydrates: 25g | Protein: 3g | Fiber: 5g | Fat: 7g | Sodium: 100mg | Sugar: 5g | Calcium: 30mg | Iron: 1mg | Potassium: 450mg

Green Bean and Potato Puree

Prep Time: 10 minutes | **Cooking Time:** 25 minutes | **Per Serving:** 4

Ingredients:

- 2 cups green beans, trimmed
- 2 medium potatoes, peeled and diced
- 1 small onion, chopped
- 2 tablespoons olive oil
- 1/2 cup low-sodium vegetable broth
- Salt and pepper, to taste

Instructions:

1. Steam green beans and potatoes until tender, about 15-20 minutes.
2. In a pan, heat olive oil and sauté onion until soft, about 5 minutes.
3. Combine green beans, potatoes, and sautéed onion in a blender.
4. Add vegetable broth and puree until smooth.
5. Season with salt and pepper to taste.
6. Serve warm.

Nutritional Information (per serving):
Calories: 140 | Carbohydrates: 30g | Protein: 4g | Fiber: 6g | Fat: 5g | Sodium: 250mg | Sugar: 5g | Calcium: 40mg | Iron: 1mg | Potassium: 600mg

Pea and Spinach Puree

Prep Time: 5 minutes | **Cooking Time:** 15 minutes | **Per Serving:** 4

Ingredients:

- 2 cups peas (fresh or frozen)
- 2 cups fresh spinach leaves
- 1/2 cup low-sodium vegetable broth
- 1 tablespoon olive oil
- Salt and pepper, to taste

Instructions:

1. Steam peas and spinach until tender, about 10 minutes.
2. Transfer peas, spinach, vegetable broth, and olive oil to a blender.
3. Puree until smooth.
4. Season with salt and pepper to taste.
5. Serve warm.

Nutritional Information (per serving):
Calories: 110 | Carbohydrates: 18g | Protein: 8g | Fiber: 7g | Fat: 4g | Sodium: 200mg | Sugar: 6g | Calcium: 40mg | Iron: 3mg | Potassium: 400mg

Garlic Mashed Parsnips

Prep Time: 10 minutes | **Cooking Time:** 20 minutes | **Per Serving:** 4

Ingredients:

- 4 large parsnips, peeled and chopped
- 3 garlic cloves, peeled
- 2 tablespoons butter or olive oil
- 1/4 cup low-sodium vegetable broth
- Salt and pepper, to taste

Instructions:

1. Steam parsnips and garlic until tender, about 20 minutes.
2. Transfer to a blender, add butter and vegetable broth.
3. Puree until smooth.
4. Season with salt and pepper to taste.
5. Serve warm.

Nutritional Information (per serving):
Calories: 130 | Carbohydrates: 28g | Protein: 3g | Fiber: 6g | Fat: 5g | Sodium: 150mg | Sugar: 6g | Calcium: 40mg | Iron: 1mg | Potassium: 500mg

Chapter 8 Snacks and Desserts

Puréed Sticky Toffee Pudding

Prep Time: 15 minutes | **Cooking Time:** 30 minutes | **Per Serving:** 4

Ingredients:

- 1 cup dates, pitted and chopped
- 1 cup boiling water
- 1 teaspoon baking soda
- 1/2 cup butter, softened
- 1/2 cup brown sugar
- 2 eggs
- 1 cup self-raising flour
- 1/2 teaspoon vanilla extract
- 1/2 cup heavy cream
- 1/2 cup brown sugar (for sauce)
- 2 tablespoons butter (for sauce)
- 1/4 cup heavy cream (for sauce)

Instructions:

1. Preheat oven to 350°F (175°C).
2. Soak dates in boiling water with baking soda for 10 minutes.
3. Cream butter and brown sugar until light and fluffy. Add eggs one at a time, then vanilla.
4. Fold in flour and soaked dates with liquid.
5. Pour batter into a greased baking dish and bake for 25-30 minutes.
6. For sauce, heat brown sugar, butter, and cream in a saucepan until smooth and thickened.
7. Blend the pudding with sauce until smooth and creamy.
8. Serve warm.

Nutritional Information (per serving):
Calories: 350 | Carbohydrates: 50g | Protein: 4g | Fiber: 3g | Fat: 15g | Sodium: 150mg | Sugar: 40g | Calcium: 80mg | Iron: 1.5mg | Potassium: 300mg

Puréed Banoffee Pie

Prep Time: 10 minutes | **Cooking Time:** 0 minutes | **Per Serving:** 4

Ingredients:

- 2 ripe bananas
- 1/2 cup dulce de leche or caramel sauce
- 1/2 cup whipped cream
- 1/2 cup crushed digestive biscuits (optional, for texture)
- 1 teaspoon vanilla extract

Instructions:

1. Blend bananas, dulce de leche, whipped cream, and vanilla until smooth.
2. If desired, add crushed biscuits and blend gently for some texture or omit for smooth puree.
3. Chill before serving.

Nutritional Information (per serving):
Calories: 300 | Carbohydrates: 45g | Protein: 3g | Fiber: 3g | Fat: 10g | Sodium: 100mg | Sugar: 35g | Calcium: 70mg | Iron: 0.5mg | Potassium: 400mg

Soft Chocolate Sponge Cake Puree

Prep Time: 15 minutes | **Cooking Time:** 25 minutes | **Per Serving:** 4

Ingredients:

- 1/2 cup all-purpose flour
- 1/4 cup cocoa powder
- 1/2 teaspoon baking powder
- 1/4 teaspoon salt
- 1/2 cup sugar
- 2 eggs
- 1/4 cup milk
- 1/4 cup vegetable oil
- 1 teaspoon vanilla extract

Instructions:

1. Preheat oven to 350°F (175°C).
2. Whisk together flour, cocoa, baking powder, and salt.
3. In another bowl, beat sugar and eggs until fluffy. Add milk, oil, and vanilla.
4. Combine wet and dry ingredients.
5. Pour batter into a greased pan and bake for 20-25 minutes.
6. Cool, then blend with a little milk until smooth puree.
7. Serve at room temperature.

Nutritional Information (per serving):
Calories: 280 | Carbohydrates: 40g | Protein: 5g | Fiber: 3g | Fat: 10g | Sodium: 150mg | Sugar: 30g | Calcium: 60mg | Iron: 2mg | Potassium: 250mg

Puréed Rice Pudding

Prep Time: 5 minutes | **Cooking Time:** 40 minutes | **Per Serving:** 4

Ingredients:

- 1/2 cup Arborio rice
- 4 cups milk (dairy or plant-based)
- 1/4 cup sugar
- 1 teaspoon vanilla extract
- 1/2 teaspoon ground cinnamon

Instructions:

1. In a saucepan, combine rice, milk, and sugar.
2. Cook over low heat, stirring frequently, until rice is very soft and pudding thickens, about 35-40 minutes.
3. Stir in vanilla and cinnamon.
4. Cool slightly, then blend until smooth.
5. Serve warm or chilled.

Nutritional Information (per serving):
Calories: 220 | Carbohydrates: 38g | Protein: 7g | Fiber: 1g | Fat: 5g | Sodium: 100mg | Sugar: 20g | Calcium: 250mg | Iron: 0.5mg | Potassium: 150mg

Puréed Apple Crumble

Prep Time: 10 minutes | **Cooking Time:** 25 minutes | **Per Serving:** 4

Ingredients:

- 4 apples, peeled, cored, and chopped
- 1/2 cup rolled oats
- 1/4 cup brown sugar
- 1/4 cup butter, softened
- 1 teaspoon ground cinnamon
- 1/4 cup water

Instructions:

1. Preheat oven to 350°F (175°C).
2. Place apples and water in a baking dish and bake for 15 minutes until soft.
3. Mix oats, brown sugar, butter, and cinnamon to make crumble topping.
4. Sprinkle topping over apples and bake for another 10 minutes.
5. Cool slightly and blend until smooth.
6. Serve warm.

Nutritional Information (per serving):
Calories: 250 | Carbohydrates: 45g | Protein: 3g | Fiber: 5g | Fat: 8g | Sodium: 50mg | Sugar: 30g | Calcium: 40mg | Iron: 1mg | Potassium: 200mg

Fresh Banana Curd Puree

Prep Time: 5 minutes | **Cooking Time:** 10 minutes | **Per Serving:** 4

Ingredients:

- 2 ripe bananas
- 2 eggs
- 1/4 cup sugar
- 1/4 cup lemon juice
- 2 tablespoons butter

Instructions:

1. In a saucepan, whisk eggs, sugar, and lemon juice.
2. Cook over low heat, stirring constantly until thickened, about 7-10 minutes.
3. Remove from heat and stir in butter until melted.
4. Cool slightly and blend with bananas until smooth.
5. Serve chilled.

Nutritional Information (per serving):
Calories: 180 | Carbohydrates: 30g | Protein: 3g | Fiber: 2g | Fat: 6g | Sodium: 30mg | Sugar: 25g | Calcium: 20mg | Iron: 0.3mg | Potassium: 350mg

Strawberry Mousse Puree

Prep Time: 10 minutes | **Cooking Time:** 0 minutes | **Per Serving:** 4

Ingredients:

- 2 cups fresh strawberries, hulled
- 1/2 cup whipped cream
- 2 tablespoons sugar
- 1 teaspoon lemon juice

Instructions:

1. Blend strawberries, sugar, and lemon juice until smooth.
2. Fold in whipped cream gently.
3. Chill before serving.

Nutritional Information (per serving):
Calories: 120 | Carbohydrates: 20g | Protein: 1g | Fiber: 3g | Fat: 5g | Sodium: 5mg | Sugar: 18g | Calcium: 30mg | Iron: 0.3mg | Potassium: 200mg

Mango Panna Cotta Puree

Prep Time: 10 minutes | **Cooking Time:** 10 minutes + chilling | **Per Serving:** 4

Ingredients:

- 1 cup mango puree (fresh or frozen mango blended)
- 1 cup heavy cream
- 1/4 cup sugar
- 1 teaspoon gelatin powder
- 2 tablespoons water

Instructions:

1. Sprinkle gelatin over water and let bloom for 5 minutes.
2. Heat cream and sugar in a saucepan until sugar dissolves. Remove from heat and stir in gelatin until dissolved.
3. Mix in mango puree.
4. Pour into serving dishes and chill for at least 4 hours until set.
5. Blend before serving if needed for puree texture.

Nutritional Information (per serving):
Calories: 250 | Carbohydrates: 20g | Protein: 3g | Fiber: 2g | Fat: 18g | Sodium: 20mg | Sugar: 18g | Calcium: 100mg | Iron: 0.3mg | Potassium: 150mg

Peanut Butter Mousse Puree

Prep Time: 10 minutes | **Cooking Time:** 0 minutes | **Per Serving:** 4

Ingredients:

- 1/2 cup smooth peanut butter
- 1/2 cup whipped cream
- 2 tablespoons honey or maple syrup
- 1/4 cup milk or plant-based milk

Instructions:

1. Blend peanut butter, honey, and milk until smooth.
2. Fold in whipped cream gently.
3. Chill before serving.

Nutritional Information (per serving):
Calories: 300 | Carbohydrates: 15g | Protein: 10g | Fiber: 3g | Fat: 25g | Sodium: 150mg | Sugar: 12g | Calcium: 40mg | Iron: 1mg | Potassium: 250mg

Peach Mousse Puree

Prep Time: 10 minutes | **Cooking Time:** 0 minutes | **Per Serving:** 4

Ingredients:

- 2 ripe peaches, peeled and chopped
- 1/2 cup whipped cream
- 2 tablespoons sugar
- 1 teaspoon lemon juice

Instructions:

1. Blend peaches, sugar, and lemon juice until smooth.
2. Fold in whipped cream gently.
3. Chill before serving.

Nutritional Information (per serving):
Calories: 130 | Carbohydrates: 22g | Protein: 1g | Fiber: 3g | Fat: 5g | Sodium: 5mg | Sugar: 18g | Calcium: 30mg | Iron: 0.3mg | Potassium: 200mg

Homemade Vanilla Pudding

Prep Time: 10 minutes | **Cooking Time:** 15 minutes | **Per Serving:** 4

Ingredients:

- 2 cups milk (dairy or plant-based)
- 1/3 cup sugar
- 3 tablespoons cornstarch
- 1/4 teaspoon salt
- 2 teaspoons vanilla extract
- 2 tablespoons butter

Instructions:

1. In a saucepan, whisk together sugar, cornstarch, and salt. Gradually whisk in milk until smooth.

2. Cook over medium heat, stirring constantly, until mixture thickens and boils, about 8-10 minutes.
3. Remove from heat and stir in butter and vanilla extract.
4. Pour into serving dishes and chill for at least 2 hours before serving.
5. Blend before serving if needed for smooth puree texture.

Nutritional Information (per serving):
Calories: 180 | Carbohydrates: 30g | Protein: 6g | Fiber: 0g | Fat: 5g | Sodium: 150mg | Sugar: 25g | Calcium: 250mg | Iron: 0.1mg | Potassium: 250mg

Passion Fruit Pudding Cake

Prep Time: 15 minutes | **Cooking Time:** 40 minutes | **Per Serving:** 4

Ingredients:

- 1 cup passion fruit pulp (fresh or frozen)
- 1/2 cup sugar
- 1/2 cup all-purpose flour
- 1/4 cup butter, softened
- 2 eggs
- 1 teaspoon baking powder

Instructions:

1. Preheat oven to 350°F (175°C).
2. Beat butter and sugar until light and fluffy. Add eggs one at a time.
3. Mix flour and baking powder; gradually add to butter mixture.
4. Fold in passion fruit pulp.
5. Pour batter into greased baking dish and bake for 35-40 minutes.
6. Cool slightly and blend until smooth for puree texture.
7. Serve warm or chilled.

Nutritional Information (per serving):
Calories: 280 | Carbohydrates: 45g | Protein: 5g | Fiber: 2g | Fat: 8g | Sodium: 150mg | Sugar: 35g | Calcium: 50mg | Iron: 1mg | Potassium: 150mg

Easy Milk Pudding

Prep Time: 5 minutes | **Cooking Time:** 20 minutes | **Per Serving:** 4

Ingredients:

- 2 cups milk (dairy or plant-based)
- 1/3 cup sugar
- 3 tablespoons cornstarch
- 1 teaspoon vanilla extract

Instructions:

1. In a saucepan, whisk sugar and cornstarch. Gradually add milk, whisking until smooth.
2. Cook over medium heat, stirring constantly, until thickened, about 15-20 minutes.
3. Remove from heat and stir in vanilla extract.
4. Pour into serving dishes and chill before serving.
5. Blend before serving if needed for smooth puree texture.

Nutritional Information (per serving):
Calories: 160 | Carbohydrates: 28g | Protein: 6g | Fiber: 0g | Fat: 3g | Sodium: 150mg | Sugar: 22g | Calcium: 250mg | Iron: 0.1mg | Potassium: 250mg

Simple Chocolate Mousse Puree

Prep Time: 10 minutes | **Cooking Time:** 0 minutes | **Per Serving:** 4

Ingredients:

- 1/2 cup dark chocolate, melted
- 1 cup heavy cream, whipped
- 2 tablespoons sugar
- 1 teaspoon vanilla extract

Instructions:

1. Fold melted chocolate into whipped cream gently.
2. Add sugar and vanilla extract, mix until combined.
3. Chill before serving.

4. Blend before serving if needed for smooth puree texture.

Nutritional Information (per serving):
Calories: 300 | Carbohydrates: 15g | Protein: 3g | Fiber: 2g | Fat: 25g | Sodium: 20mg | Sugar: 12g | Calcium: 40mg | Iron: 2mg | Potassium: 150mg

Raspberry Sorbet Puree

Prep Time: 5 minutes | **Cooking Time:** 0 minutes | **Per Serving:** 4

Ingredients:

- 3 cups fresh or frozen raspberries
- 1/4 cup sugar
- 1 tablespoon lemon juice

Instructions:

1. Blend raspberries, sugar, and lemon juice until smooth.
2. Strain to remove seeds if desired.
3. Freeze for 1-2 hours or serve immediately as a puree.

Nutritional Information (per serving):
Calories: 80 | Carbohydrates: 18g | Protein: 1g | Fiber: 4g | Fat: 0g | Sodium: 0mg | Sugar: 15g | Calcium: 20mg | Iron: 0.5mg | Potassium: 150mg

Ube Halaya Puree

Prep Time: 10 minutes | **Cooking Time:** 45 minutes | **Per Serving:** 4

Ingredients:

- 2 cups grated purple yam (ube)
- 1 cup coconut milk
- 1/2 cup condensed milk
- 1/4 cup sugar
- 2 tablespoons butter

Instructions:

1. In a pot, combine grated ube, coconut milk, condensed milk, and sugar.
2. Cook over medium heat, stirring constantly until thickened, about 40 minutes.
3. Stir in butter until melted.
4. Cool slightly and blend until smooth.
5. Serve warm or chilled.

Nutritional Information (per serving):
Calories: 280 | Carbohydrates: 50g | Protein: 3g | Fiber: 4g | Fat: 8g | Sodium: 50mg | Sugar: 40g | Calcium: 40mg | Iron: 1mg | Potassium: 300mg

Pots de Crème Puree

Prep Time: 10 minutes | **Cooking Time:** 40 minutes | **Per Serving:** 4

Ingredients:

- 2 cups heavy cream
- 4 egg yolks
- 1/2 cup sugar
- 1 teaspoon vanilla extract

Instructions:

1. Preheat oven to 325°F (160°C).
2. Heat cream until just simmering.
3. Whisk egg yolks and sugar until pale.
4. Gradually whisk hot cream into egg mixture.
5. Stir in vanilla extract.
6. Pour into ramekins and bake in a water bath for 30-35 minutes until set.
7. Cool and blend until smooth if needed.
8. Chill before serving.

Nutritional Information (per serving):
Calories: 350 | Carbohydrates: 25g | Protein: 6g | Fiber: 0g | Fat: 25g | Sodium: 50mg | Sugar: 25g | Calcium: 100mg | Iron: 0.1mg | Potassium: 150mg

Creamy Mango Pudding

Prep Time: 10 minutes | **Cooking Time:** 10 minutes | **Per Serving:** 4

Ingredients:

- 1 cup mango puree
- 1 cup heavy cream
- 1/4 cup sugar
- 1 teaspoon gelatin powder
- 2 tablespoons water

Instructions:

1. Bloom gelatin in water for 5 minutes.
2. Heat cream and sugar until sugar dissolves. Remove from heat and stir in gelatin until dissolved.
3. Mix in mango puree.
4. Pour into serving dishes and chill until set, about 4 hours.
5. Blend before serving if needed.

Nutritional Information (per serving):
Calories: 250 | Carbohydrates: 20g | Protein: 3g | Fiber: 2g | Fat: 18g | Sodium: 20mg | Sugar: 18g | Calcium: 100mg | Iron: 0.3mg | Potassium: 150mg

Coconut Rice Pudding Puree

Prep Time: 5 minutes | **Cooking Time:** 40 minutes | **Per Serving:** 4

Ingredients:

- 1/2 cup Arborio rice
- 4 cups coconut milk
- 1/4 cup sugar
- 1 teaspoon vanilla extract

Instructions:

1. Combine rice, coconut milk, and sugar in a saucepan.
2. Cook over low heat, stirring frequently, until rice is very soft and pudding thickens, about 35-40 minutes.
3. Stir in vanilla extract.
4. Cool slightly and blend until smooth.
5. Serve warm or chilled.

Nutritional Information (per serving):
Calories: 280 | Carbohydrates: 40g | Protein: 5g | Fiber: 1g | Fat: 12g | Sodium: 50mg | Sugar: 20g | Calcium: 40mg | Iron: 0.5mg | Potassium: 150mg

Lemon Custard Puree

Prep Time: 10 minutes | **Cooking Time:** 15 minutes | **Per Serving:** 4

Ingredients:

- 2 cups milk (dairy or plant-based)
- 3 eggs
- 1/2 cup sugar
- 1/4 cup lemon juice
- Zest of 1 lemon

Instructions:

1. In a saucepan, heat milk until warm.
2. In a bowl, whisk eggs, sugar, lemon juice, and zest.
3. Slowly whisk warm milk into egg mixture.
4. Return mixture to saucepan and cook over low heat, stirring constantly until thickened, about 10-15 minutes.
5. Cool slightly and blend until smooth.
6. Chill before serving.

Nutritional Information (per serving):
Calories: 200 | Carbohydrates: 25g | Protein: 7g | Fiber: 0g | Fat: 5g | Sodium: 100mg | Sugar: 20g | Calcium: 250mg | Iron: 0.1mg | Potassium: 250mg

Chapter 9 Bonus 1

Allergy Friendly and Special Diet Recipes

Dairy-Free Pumpkin and Sweet Potato Puree

Prep Time: 10 minutes | **Cooking Time:** 25 minutes | **Per Serving:** 4

Ingredients:

- 1 cup pumpkin, peeled and cubed
- 1 cup sweet potato, peeled and diced
- 1/2 cup water or unsweetened almond milk
- 1 tablespoon olive oil
- 1/2 teaspoon ground cinnamon
- Pinch of salt

Instructions:

1. Steam pumpkin and sweet potato until tender, about 20-25 minutes.
2. Transfer to a blender, add water or almond milk, olive oil, cinnamon, and salt.
3. Puree until smooth and creamy.
4. Serve warm.

Nutritional Information (per serving):
Calories: 120 | Carbohydrates: 28g | Protein: 2g | Fiber: 5g | Fat: 5g | Sodium: 50mg | Sugar: 7g | Calcium: 40mg | Iron: 1mg | Potassium: 450mg

Gluten-Free Carrot and Apple Puree

Prep Time: 10 minutes | **Cooking Time:** 20 minutes | **Per Serving:** 4

Ingredients:

- 3 large carrots, peeled and chopped
- 2 apples, peeled, cored, and chopped
- 1/4 cup water
- 1/2 teaspoon ground cinnamon

Instructions:

1. Steam carrots and apples until tender, about 20 minutes.
2. Transfer to a blender, add water and cinnamon.
3. Puree until smooth.
4. Serve warm or chilled.

Nutritional Information (per serving):
Calories: 110 | Carbohydrates: 28g | Protein: 1g | Fiber: 5g | Fat: 0g | Sodium: 10mg | Sugar: 15g | Calcium: 30mg | Iron: 0.5mg | Potassium: 400mg

Nut-Free Banana and Oat Smoothie

Prep Time: 5 minutes | **Cooking Time:** 0 minutes | **Per Serving:** 1

Ingredients:

- 1 ripe banana
- 1/2 cup rolled oats
- 1 cup oat milk or other nut-free milk alternative
- 1 teaspoon honey or maple syrup (optional)
- 1/2 teaspoon ground cinnamon

Instructions:

1. Combine all ingredients in a blender.
2. Blend until smooth and creamy.
3. Serve immediately.

Nutritional Information (per serving):
Calories: 250 | Carbohydrates: 50g | Protein: 5g | Fiber: 6g | Fat: 2g | Sodium: 50mg | Sugar: 18g | Calcium: 150mg | Iron: 1mg | Potassium: 450mg

Soy-Free Lentil and Vegetable Puree

Prep Time: 10 minutes | **Cooking Time:** 30 minutes | **Per Serving:** 4

Ingredients:

- 1 cup red lentils, rinsed
- 2 carrots, peeled and chopped
- 1 zucchini, chopped
- 1 small onion, chopped
- 4 cups low-sodium vegetable broth
- 1 tablespoon olive oil
- 1/2 teaspoon ground cumin
- Salt and pepper, to taste

Instructions:

1. Heat olive oil in a pot over medium heat. Add onion and sauté until soft, about 5 minutes.
2. Add carrots, zucchini, lentils, cumin, and vegetable broth. Bring to a boil.
3. Reduce heat and simmer for 20-25 minutes until lentils and vegetables are tender.
4. Puree until smooth.
5. Season with salt and pepper to taste.
6. Serve warm.

Nutritional Information (per serving):
Calories: 180 | Carbohydrates: 30g | Protein: 12g | Fiber: 8g | Fat: 5g | Sodium: 320mg | Sugar: 7g | Calcium: 40mg | Iron: 3mg | Potassium: 500mg

Egg-Free Chickpea and Spinach Puree

Prep Time: 10 minutes | **Cooking Time:** 20 minutes | **Per Serving:** 4

Ingredients:

- 1 can (15 oz) chickpeas, drained and rinsed
- 2 cups fresh spinach leaves
- 1 small onion, chopped
- 2 garlic cloves, minced
- 2 tablespoons olive oil
- 1/2 cup low-sodium vegetable broth
- Salt and pepper, to taste

Instructions:

1. Heat olive oil in a pot over medium heat. Add onion and garlic; sauté until soft, about 5 minutes.
2. Add chickpeas, spinach, and vegetable broth. Cook until spinach is wilted and chickpeas are soft, about 10-15 minutes.
3. Puree until smooth.
4. Season with salt and pepper to taste.
5. Serve warm.

Nutritional Information (per serving):
Calories: 200 | Carbohydrates: 30g | Protein: 10g | Fiber: 8g | Fat: 7g | Sodium: 250mg | Sugar: 5g | Calcium: 80mg | Iron: 4mg | Potassium: 600mg

Low-Sodium Pureed Cauliflower and Pea Soup

Prep Time: 10 minutes | **Cooking Time:** 20 minutes | **Per Serving:** 4

Ingredients:

- 1 head cauliflower, cut into florets
- 2 cups peas (fresh or frozen)
- 1 small onion, chopped
- 4 cups water or low-sodium vegetable broth
- 1 tablespoon olive oil
- Salt and pepper, to taste (use sparingly)

Instructions:

1. Heat olive oil in a pot over medium heat. Add onion and sauté until soft, about 5 minutes.
2. Add cauliflower, peas, and water or broth. Bring to a boil, then reduce heat and simmer until vegetables are tender, about 15 minutes.
3. Puree soup until smooth.
4. Season with salt and pepper sparingly.

5. Serve warm.

Nutritional Information (per serving):
Calories: 110 | Carbohydrates: 20g | Protein: 7g | Fiber: 7g | Fat: 4g | Sodium: 100mg | Sugar: 6g | Calcium: 40mg | Iron: 2mg | Potassium: 400mg

Sugar-Free Cinnamon Apple Puree

Prep Time: 10 minutes | **Cooking Time:** 20 minutes | **Per Serving:** 4

Ingredients:

- 4 apples, peeled, cored, and chopped
- 1/2 teaspoon ground cinnamon
- 1/4 cup water

Instructions:

1. Steam apples with water until tender, about 20 minutes.
2. Transfer to a blender, add cinnamon, and puree until smooth.
3. Serve warm or chilled.

Nutritional Information (per serving):
Calories: 90 | Carbohydrates: 24g | Protein: 0g | Fiber: 4g | Fat: 0g | Sodium: 0mg | Sugar: 19g | Calcium: 20mg | Iron: 0.3mg | Potassium: 150mg

Vegan Sweet Potato and Coconut Puree

Prep Time: 10 minutes | **Cooking Time:** 25 minutes | **Per Serving:** 4

Ingredients:

- 2 medium sweet potatoes, peeled and diced
- 1 cup coconut milk (full fat)
- 1/2 teaspoon ground cinnamon
- 1 tablespoon maple syrup (optional)
- Pinch of salt

Instructions:

1. Steam sweet potatoes until tender, about 20-25 minutes.
2. Transfer to a blender, add coconut milk, cinnamon, maple syrup (if using), and salt.
3. Puree until smooth and creamy.
4. Serve warm.

Nutritional Information (per serving):
Calories: 150 | Carbohydrates: 30g | Protein: 2g | Fiber: 4g | Fat: 6g | Sodium: 50mg | Sugar: 8g | Calcium: 40mg | Iron: 1mg | Potassium: 450mg

Gluten-Free Zucchini and Basil Puree

Prep Time: 10 minutes | **Cooking Time:** 15 minutes | **Per Serving:** 4

Ingredients:

- 3 medium zucchinis, chopped
- 1/4 cup fresh basil leaves
- 1/2 cup low-sodium vegetable broth
- 1 tablespoon olive oil
- Salt and pepper, to taste

Instructions:

1. Steam zucchini until tender, about 10-12 minutes.
2. Transfer zucchini, basil, vegetable broth, and olive oil to a blender.
3. Puree until smooth.
4. Season with salt and pepper to taste.
5. Serve warm.

Nutritional Information (per serving):
Calories: 90 | Carbohydrates: 15g | Protein: 3g | Fiber: 4g | Fat: 5g | Sodium: 150mg | Sugar: 7g | Calcium: 40mg | Iron: 1mg | Potassium: 450mg

Dairy-Free Creamy Butternut Squash Puree

Prep Time: 10 minutes | **Cooking Time:** 30 minutes | **Per Serving:** 4

Ingredients:

- 1 medium butternut squash, peeled and cubed
- 1 cup coconut milk (full fat)
- 1 tablespoon olive oil
- Salt and pepper, to taste

Instructions:

1. Steam butternut squash until tender, about 25-30 minutes.
2. Transfer to a blender, add coconut milk, olive oil, salt, and pepper.
3. Puree until smooth and creamy.
4. Serve warm.

Nutritional Information (per serving):
Calories: 160 | Carbohydrates: 25g | Protein: 3g | Fiber: 5g | Fat: 7g | Sodium: 100mg | Sugar: 5g | Calcium: 30mg | Iron: 1mg | Potassium: 450mg

Allergy-Friendly Creamy Pea and Mint Puree

Prep Time: 5 minutes | **Cooking Time:** 15 minutes | **Per Serving:** 4

Ingredients:

- 3 cups fresh or frozen peas
- 1/4 cup fresh mint leaves
- 1/2 cup water or low-sodium vegetable broth
- 1 tablespoon olive oil
- Salt and pepper, to taste

Instructions:

1. Steam peas until tender, about 10 minutes.
2. Transfer peas, mint, water or broth, and olive oil to a blender.
3. Puree until smooth.
4. Season with salt and pepper to taste.
5. Serve warm.

Nutritional Information (per serving):
Calories: 110 | Carbohydrates: 20g | Protein: 7g | Fiber: 6g | Fat: 4g | Sodium: 200mg | Sugar: 6g | Calcium: 40mg | Iron: 2mg | Potassium: 350mg

Nut-Free Roasted Carrot and Parsnip Puree

Prep Time: 10 minutes | **Cooking Time:** 30 minutes | **Per Serving:** 4

Ingredients:

- 3 large carrots, peeled and chopped
- 3 large parsnips, peeled and chopped
- 2 tablespoons olive oil
- 1/2 cup water or low-sodium vegetable broth
- Salt and pepper, to taste

Instructions:

1. Preheat oven to 400°F (200°C).
2. Toss carrots and parsnips with olive oil, salt, and pepper.
3. Roast on a baking sheet for 25-30 minutes until tender and caramelized.
4. Transfer to a blender, add water or broth, and puree until smooth.
5. Serve warm.

Nutritional Information (per serving):
Calories: 130 | Carbohydrates: 28g | Protein: 3g | Fiber: 6g | Fat: 5g | Sodium: 150mg | Sugar: 8g | Calcium: 40mg | Iron: 1mg | Potassium: 500mg

Soy-Free Sweet Corn and Potato Puree

Prep Time: 10 minutes | **Cooking Time:** 25 minutes | **Per Serving:** 4

Ingredients:

- 3 cups corn kernels (fresh or frozen)
- 2 medium potatoes, peeled and diced
- 1 small onion, chopped
- 2 tablespoons olive oil
- 1/2 cup water or low-sodium vegetable broth
- Salt and pepper, to taste

Instructions:

1. Steam corn and potatoes until tender, about 20-25 minutes.
2. In a pan, heat olive oil and sauté onion until soft, about 5 minutes.
3. Combine corn, potatoes, sautéed onion, and water or broth in a blender.
4. Puree until smooth.
5. Season with salt and pepper to taste.
6. Serve warm.

Nutritional Information (per serving):
Calories: 160 | Carbohydrates: 35g | Protein: 5g | Fiber: 5g | Fat: 5g | Sodium: 150mg | Sugar: 8g | Calcium: 50mg | Iron: 1mg | Potassium: 500mg

Egg-Free Pumpkin and Sage Puree

Prep Time: 10 minutes | **Cooking Time:** 30 minutes | **Per Serving:** 4

Ingredients:

- 1 medium pumpkin, peeled and cubed
- 1 tablespoon fresh sage, chopped (or 1 teaspoon dried sage)
- 2 tablespoons olive oil
- 1/2 cup water or low-sodium vegetable broth
- Salt and pepper, to taste

Instructions:

1. Preheat oven to 400°F (200°C).
2. Toss pumpkin with olive oil, sage, salt, and pepper.
3. Roast for 25-30 minutes until tender.
4. Transfer to a blender, add water or broth, and puree until smooth.
5. Serve warm.

Nutritional Information (per serving):
Calories: 140 | Carbohydrates: 28g | Protein: 2g | Fiber: 5g | Fat: 6g | Sodium: 150mg | Sugar: 7g | Calcium: 40mg | Iron: 0.8mg | Potassium: 450mg

Low-FODMAP Pureed Pumpkin and Carrot Soup

Prep Time: 10 minutes | **Cooking Time:** 30 minutes | **Per Serving:** 4

Ingredients:

- 1 cup pumpkin, peeled and cubed
- 2 large carrots, peeled and chopped
- 1 tablespoon garlic-infused olive oil (FODMAP friendly)
- 4 cups low-sodium vegetable broth (FODMAP friendly)
- Salt and pepper, to taste

Instructions:

1. Heat garlic-infused olive oil in a pot over medium heat.
2. Add pumpkin and carrots; sauté for 5 minutes.
3. Add vegetable broth and bring to a boil.
4. Reduce heat and simmer for 20-25 minutes until vegetables are tender.
5. Puree until smooth.
6. Season with salt and pepper to taste.
7. Serve warm.

Nutritional Information (per serving):
Calories: 120 | Carbohydrates: 28g | Protein: 2g | Fiber: 6g | Fat: 5g | Sodium: 150mg | Sugar: 8g | Calcium: 40mg | Iron: 1mg | Potassium: 450mg

Vegan Roasted Beet and Apple Puree

Prep Time: 10 minutes | **Cooking Time:** 30 minutes | **Per Serving:** 4

Ingredients:

- 2 medium beets, peeled and chopped
- 2 apples, peeled, cored, and chopped
- 2 tablespoons olive oil
- 1/4 cup water or low-sodium vegetable broth
- Salt and pepper, to taste

Instructions:

1. Preheat oven to 400°F (200°C).
2. Toss beets and apples with olive oil, salt, and pepper.
3. Roast for 25-30 minutes until tender.
4. Transfer to a blender, add water or broth, and puree until smooth.
5. Serve warm.

Nutritional Information (per serving):
Calories: 140 | Carbohydrates: 32g | Protein: 2g | Fiber: 6g | Fat: 7g | Sodium: 50mg | Sugar: 18g | Calcium: 40mg | Iron: 1.2mg | Potassium: 600mg

Gluten-Free Creamy Broccoli and Cauliflower Puree

Prep Time: 10 minutes | **Cooking Time:** 20 minutes | **Per Serving:** 4

Ingredients:

- 2 cups broccoli florets
- 2 cups cauliflower florets
- 1/2 cup coconut milk (or dairy-free milk)
- 1 tablespoon olive oil
- Salt and pepper, to taste

Instructions:

1. Steam broccoli and cauliflower until tender, about 15-20 minutes.
2. Transfer to a blender, add coconut milk, olive oil, salt, and pepper.
3. Puree until smooth and creamy.
4. Serve warm.

Nutritional Information (per serving):
Calories: 130 | Carbohydrates: 15g | Protein: 5g | Fiber: 6g | Fat: 7g | Sodium: 150mg | Sugar: 5g | Calcium: 60mg | Iron: 1.5mg | Potassium: 500mg

Dairy-Free Spinach and Potato Puree

Prep Time: 10 minutes | **Cooking Time:** 25 minutes | **Per Serving:** 4

Ingredients:

- 2 cups fresh spinach leaves
- 3 medium potatoes, peeled and diced
- 1/2 cup coconut milk (or other dairy-free milk)
- 1 tablespoon olive oil
- Salt and pepper, to taste

Instructions:

1. Steam spinach and potatoes until tender, about 20-25 minutes.
2. Transfer to a blender, add coconut milk and olive oil.
3. Puree until smooth.
4. Season with salt and pepper to taste.
5. Serve warm.

Nutritional Information (per serving):
Calories: 140 | Carbohydrates: 30g | Protein: 5g | Fiber: 6g | Fat: 6g | Sodium: 150mg | Sugar: 5g | Calcium: 80mg | Iron: 2mg | Potassium: 600mg

Nut-Free Sweet Potato and Apple Mash

Prep Time: 10 minutes | **Cooking Time:** 25 minutes | **Per Serving:** 4

Ingredients:

- 2 medium sweet potatoes, peeled and diced
- 2 apples, peeled, cored, and chopped
- 1/4 cup water or low-sodium vegetable broth
- 1 tablespoon olive oil
- 1/2 teaspoon ground cinnamon
- Pinch of salt

Instructions:

1. Steam sweet potatoes and apples until tender, about 20-25 minutes.
2. Transfer to a blender, add water or broth, olive oil, cinnamon, and salt.
3. Puree until smooth and creamy.
4. Serve warm.

Nutritional Information (per serving):
Calories: 130 | Carbohydrates: 30g | Protein: 2g | Fiber: 5g | Fat: 5g | Sodium: 40mg | Sugar: 15g | Calcium: 40mg | Iron: 1mg | Potassium: 450mg

Soy-Free Creamy Lentil and Carrot Puree

Prep Time: 10 minutes | **Cooking Time:** 25 minutes | **Per Serving:** 4

Ingredients:

- 1 cup red lentils, rinsed
- 3 large carrots, peeled and chopped
- 1 small onion, chopped
- 2 tablespoons olive oil
- 4 cups low-sodium vegetable broth
- 1/2 teaspoon ground cumin
- Salt and pepper, to taste

Instructions:

1. Heat olive oil in a pot over medium heat. Add onion and sauté until soft, about 5 minutes.
2. Add carrots, lentils, cumin, and vegetable broth. Bring to a boil.
3. Reduce heat and simmer for 20 minutes until lentils and carrots are tender.
4. Puree until smooth.
5. Season with salt and pepper to taste.
6. Serve warm.

Nutritional Information (per serving):
Calories: 180 | Carbohydrates: 30g | Protein: 12g | Fiber: 8g | Fat: 5g | Sodium: 320mg | Sugar: 7g | Calcium: 40mg | Iron: 3mg | Potassium: 500mg

Egg-Free Roasted Red Pepper and Tomato Puree

Prep Time: 10 minutes | **Cooking Time:** 30 minutes | **Per Serving:** 4

Ingredients:

- 3 red bell peppers, halved and seeded
- 4 large tomatoes, halved
- 1 medium onion, quartered
- 3 garlic cloves, peeled
- 2 tablespoons olive oil
- 2 cups low-sodium vegetable broth
- 1 teaspoon smoked paprika
- Salt and pepper, to taste
- Fresh basil, for garnish (optional)

Instructions:

1. Preheat oven to 425°F (220°C).
2. Arrange peppers, tomatoes, onion, and garlic on a baking sheet. Drizzle with olive oil and season with salt and pepper.
3. Roast for 25-30 minutes until vegetables are soft and slightly charred.

4. Transfer to a blender, add broth and smoked paprika, and puree until smooth.
5. Heat gently if needed.
6. Serve warm, garnished with fresh basil if desired.

Nutritional Information (per serving):
Calories: 110 | Carbohydrates: 20g | Protein: 3g | Fiber: 5g | Fat: 4g | Sodium: 260mg | Sugar: 10g | Calcium: 40mg | Iron: 1mg | Potassium: 700mg

Low-Sodium Pureed Green Bean and Potato Medley

Prep Time: 10 minutes | **Cooking Time:** 25 minutes | **Per Serving:** 4

Ingredients:

- 2 cups green beans, trimmed
- 2 medium potatoes, peeled and diced
- 1 small onion, chopped
- 2 tablespoons olive oil
- 1/2 cup water
- Salt and pepper, to taste (use sparingly)

Instructions:

1. Steam green beans and potatoes until tender, about 15-20 minutes.
2. In a pan, heat olive oil and sauté onion until soft, about 5 minutes.
3. Combine green beans, potatoes, sautéed onion, and water in a blender.
4. Puree until smooth.
5. Season with salt and pepper sparingly.
6. Serve warm.

Nutritional Information (per serving):
Calories: 140 | Carbohydrates: 30g | Protein: 4g | Fiber: 6g | Fat: 5g | Sodium: 50mg | Sugar: 5g | Calcium: 40mg | Iron: 1mg | Potassium: 600mg

Vegan Pumpkin and Cinnamon Puree

Prep Time: 10 minutes | **Cooking Time:** 25 minutes | **Per Serving:** 4

Ingredients:

- 2 cups pumpkin, peeled and cubed
- 1/2 teaspoon ground cinnamon
- 1/4 cup water or low-sodium vegetable broth
- 1 tablespoon maple syrup (optional)
- Pinch of salt

Instructions:

1. Steam pumpkin until tender, about 20-25 minutes.
2. Transfer pumpkin to a blender, add cinnamon, water or broth, maple syrup (if using), and salt.
3. Puree until smooth and creamy.
4. Serve warm.

Nutritional Information (per serving):
Calories: 110 | Carbohydrates: 26g | Protein: 2g | Fiber: 5g | Fat: 0g | Sodium: 50mg | Sugar: 8g | Calcium: 40mg | Iron: 1mg | Potassium: 400mg

Gluten-Free Carrot and Ginger Puree

Prep Time: 10 minutes | **Cooking Time:** 25 minutes | **Per Serving:** 4

Ingredients:

- 5 large carrots, peeled and chopped
- 1 tablespoon fresh ginger, grated
- 1/2 cup water or low-sodium vegetable broth
- 1 tablespoon olive oil
- Salt and pepper, to taste

Instructions:

1. Steam carrots until tender, about 20 minutes.
2. Transfer carrots, ginger, water or broth, and olive oil to a blender.
3. Puree until smooth.
4. Season with salt and pepper to taste.
5. Serve warm.

Nutritional Information (per serving):
Calories: 120 | Carbohydrates: 26g | Protein: 2g | Fiber: 5g | Fat: 4g | Sodium: 150mg | Sugar: 12g | Calcium: 50mg | Iron: 0.5mg | Potassium: 600mg

Allergy-Friendly Sweet Pea and Potato Puree

Prep Time: 10 minutes | **Cooking Time:** 20 minutes | **Per Serving:** 4

Ingredients:

- 2 cups peas (fresh or frozen)
- 2 medium potatoes, peeled and diced
- 1 tablespoon olive oil
- 1/2 cup water or low-sodium vegetable broth
- Salt and pepper, to taste

Instructions:

1. Steam peas and potatoes until tender, about 15-20 minutes.
2. Transfer to a blender, add olive oil and water or broth.
3. Puree until smooth.
4. Season with salt and pepper to taste.
5. Serve warm.

Nutritional Information (per serving):
Calories: 130 | Carbohydrates: 28g | Protein: 6g | Fiber: 6g | Fat: 5g | Sodium: 50mg | Sugar: 6g | Calcium: 40mg | Iron: 2mg | Potassium: 500mg

Chapter 10: Bonus 2

Swallowing Exercises

Improving Swallowing Through Tongue-Strengthening Exercises

Exercises designed to strengthen the tongue can enhance your swallowing ability. With consistent practice, these exercises may increase both the strength and flexibility of your tongue, which can lead to better swallowing function. When combined with other swallowing exercises, they can be particularly effective.

Before swallowing, food is chewed until it reaches a manageable size and texture. During swallowing, the chewed food moves from the mouth into the pharynx, a section of the throat. From there, it travels down the esophagus, a long muscular tube, before entering the stomach and continuing through the digestive system.

This process relies on a well-coordinated effort of multiple muscles along this pathway. If any part of this muscular coordination is impaired, swallowing difficulties can occur. Weakness in these muscles may hinder the proper movement of food. Swallowing exercises aim to improve muscle strength, range of motion, and control, which can gradually restore normal swallowing function.

A speech-language pathologist (SLP) often recommends specific exercises tailored to your unique swallowing challenges. For example, if difficulties arise during the initial phase of swallowing-before the food leaves your mouth-exercises targeting muscles in the cheeks, tongue, and lips may be beneficial. Tongue-strengthening exercises, in particular, can help improve your ability to manipulate food within the mouth and propel it toward the pharynx.

If the swallowing issue occurs later in the process, your SLP might suggest different exercises focused on those stages.

These exercises can usually be performed independently at home or in a hospital setting, though some individuals may require guidance and support from healthcare professionals during practice.

Why Might Tongue-Strengthening Exercises Be Necessary?

You may be advised to do tongue-strengthening exercises if you experience difficulty swallowing, a condition known as dysphagia.

Dysphagia can cause food or liquids to mistakenly enter the airways or lungs, a problem called aspiration. Aspiration is serious because it can lead to infections like pneumonia and other complications. Early diagnosis and treatment of dysphagia are essential.

As part of managing dysphagia, your healthcare provider and speech-language pathologist (SLP) might recommend swallowing exercises, including those that focus on strengthening the tongue. These exercises are often combined with other treatments such as modifying your diet, adjusting your eating posture, medications, or sometimes surgery. Over time, these exercises help build the strength of the muscles involved in swallowing, which can improve your ability to swallow safely and reduce the risk of aspiration.

Various medical conditions can cause swallowing difficulties, including:

- Stroke
- Dementia
- Head and neck cancers

- Head injuries
- Disorders that reduce saliva production, like Sjögren's syndrome
- Neurological diseases such as Parkinson's disease
- Muscular dystrophies
- Obstructions in the esophagus, such as tumors or strictures
- Previous treatments like radiation or chemotherapy to the neck or throat

Tongue-strengthening exercises are particularly useful when the problem lies in the initial phase of swallowing, before food leaves the mouth. For example, people who have had a stroke or have dementia may benefit from these exercises to improve tongue control and movement.

Are Tongue-Strengthening Exercises Safe?

Generally, tongue-strengthening and other swallowing exercises are safe. If you experience any pain or discomfort while doing them, stop and inform your healthcare provider or therapist immediately. It is important to only perform these exercises when they have been specifically prescribed for your condition.

Preparing for Tongue-Strengthening Exercises

Before starting, you might need to adjust your posture or positioning as advised by your SLP. For instance, it might be recommended to do the exercises while sitting up rather than lying down.

To get the most benefit, perform the exercises in a quiet environment without distractions, such as turning off the TV and choosing a time when you won't be interrupted. Your SLP will provide detailed instructions tailored to your needs and let you know if any other preparation is necessary.

What Happens During Tongue-Strengthening Exercises?

Your speech-language pathologist (SLP) will guide you through specific exercises tailored to your needs and will explain how frequently you should perform them. For example, some common exercises might include:

- **Tongue Push Against a Flat Object:**
  Extend your tongue fully. Place a flat item, such as a spoon or tongue depressor, on your tongue. Press your tongue tip firmly against the object and hold for a few seconds. Repeat this five times.

- **Tongue Push from Below:**
  Repeat the previous exercise, but this time position the spoon or depressor underneath your tongue. Perform five repetitions.

- **Side-to-Side Tongue Push:**
  Stretch your tongue toward one corner of your mouth while pushing against the depressor. Hold for a few seconds, relax, then repeat on the opposite side. Complete five repetitions.

- **Tongue Curl and Extension:**
  Extend your tongue to touch the ridged area just behind your upper front teeth. Then curl your tongue backward as far as possible. Hold for a few seconds and repeat five times.

Your SLP may also recommend additional exercises aimed at strengthening the base of your tongue and enhancing your swallowing ability, such as:

- **Super-Supraglottic Swallow:**
  Take a deep breath and hold it tightly. Bear down as if having a bowel movement while swallowing, maintaining breath hold throughout. Repeat several times.

- **Gargling Simulation:**
  Pretend to gargle while pulling your tongue back as far as possible. Repeat the movement.

- **Yawning Simulation:**
  Mimic a yawn while keeping your tongue retracted as far back as you can. Repeat.

- **Dry Swallow:**
  Perform a swallow without any food or liquid, squeezing all swallowing muscles tightly, as if swallowing a pill whole. Repeat multiple times.

Usually, tongue exercises are combined with other swallowing exercises targeting muscles in the cheeks and lips. It's helpful to perform these exercises in the same sequence each time to ensure no steps are missed. Your healthcare team will design a program that addresses the specific cause of your swallowing difficulties.

Your SLP will provide detailed instructions on how to perform each exercise and how often to practice them. Typically, exercises are done multiple times daily for optimal results.

What Happens After Tongue-Strengthening Exercises?

You can return to your regular activities immediately after completing your exercises.

Keeping a log of your exercise sessions is beneficial. Recording what exercises you did, when you did them, and any difficulties you experienced helps you stay on track and provides valuable information for your SLP to monitor your progress.

Your healthcare team may adjust your exercise plan based on your improvement. Progress is often assessed through bedside swallowing evaluations or more advanced imaging techniques like fiberoptic endoscopic evaluation of swallowing (FEES) or modified barium swallow studies (MBSS). It may take several weeks before you notice significant changes.

As your swallowing function improves, your risk of aspiration decreases. This may allow your SLP to recommend changes in your diet, enabling you to safely eat a wider variety of foods. Better nutrition can enhance your overall health and quality of life.

Consistent practice of all prescribed swallowing exercises is important. Missing sessions can slow your progress. Collaborate closely with your healthcare team to ensure the best possible outcome for your swallowing health.

Key Exercises to Improve Swallowing

Swallowing Exercises: Verbal Instructions

1. Effortful Swallow

- Sit up straight.
- Collect all the saliva in your mouth onto the center of your tongue.
- Keep your lips closed tightly.
- Pretend you are swallowing a whole grape in one big, hard swallow.
- Repeat 5 to 10 times, or as directed by your therapist.

- Rest briefly between sets and repeat as often as recommended.

2. Mendelsohn Maneuver

- Place your middle three fingers gently on your Adam's apple (the front of your neck beneath your chin).
- Swallow once and feel your Adam's apple move upward.
- Swallow again, and when your Adam's apple reaches its highest point, hold it there by squeezing your throat muscles.
- Hold for as long as you can or as directed (usually a few seconds).
- Relax and repeat several times.

3. Masako Maneuver (Tongue-Hold Swallow)

- Stick out your tongue slightly.
- Gently hold your tongue between your teeth.
- Swallow while keeping your tongue held in place.
- Repeat several times.
- Do not perform this exercise with food or liquids.

4. Shaker Exercise

- Lie flat on your back.
- Lift your head to look at your toes without lifting your shoulders.
- Hold this position for a few seconds, then lower your head.
- Repeat 30 times, rest, and repeat as directed.

5. Supraglottic Swallow

- Take a deep breath and hold it tightly.
- Swallow while holding your breath.
- Immediately after swallowing, cough to clear your throat.
- Repeat several times.

6. Super-Supraglottic Swallow

- Inhale and hold your breath very tightly.
- Bear down as if having a bowel movement.
- Keep holding your breath and bearing down as you swallow.
- Repeat a few times.
- *Note:* Avoid if you have uncontrolled blood pressure.

7. Tongue Range of Motion Exercises

- Extend your tongue to touch the bumpy ridge behind your upper front teeth.
- Then curl your tongue backward as far as possible.
- Hold for a few seconds.
- Repeat 5 times.
- Also, extend your tongue to the corners of your mouth, pushing against an object if available, holding for a few seconds, then relaxing. Repeat on both sides.

8. Dry Swallow

- Swallow without food or liquid, squeezing all your swallowing muscles as tightly as possible.
- Imagine swallowing a pill whole.
- Repeat several times.

9. Yawn and Gargle Simulations

- Pretend to yawn while holding your tongue back as far as possible. Repeat.
- Pretend to gargle while holding your tongue back as far as possible. Repeat.

Tips for Practice

- Perform these exercises as instructed by your speech-language pathologist (SLP).
- Practice several times a day for the best results.
- Keep a log of your exercises and any difficulties.
- Perform exercises in a quiet, distraction-free environment.
- Always follow your healthcare provider's guidance and report any pain or discomfort.

Important Notes

- These exercises should be performed under the guidance of a speech-language pathologist or healthcare professional to ensure correct technique and safety.
- Some exercises are contraindicated in cases of cognitive impairment, neck problems, or tongue weakness.
- Repetitions, sets, and duration vary per individual and should be customized by a clinician.

Chapter 11

Meal Plan

Day	Breakfast	Lunch	Dinner	Dessert
1	Cinnamon Roll Breakfast Smoothie (26)	Creamy Roasted Cauliflower Soup (34)	Pureed Chicken and Vegetable Medley (50)	Puréed Sticky Toffee Pudding (68)
2	Mango + Kale Baby Food Puree with Ginger (27)	SheetPan Tomato Soup (34)	Pureed Beef and Root Vegetable Stew (52)	Puréed Banoffee Pie (68)
3	Roasted Pear + Date Baby Food Puree (28)	Creamy Corn Soup with Jalapeños (35)	Pureed Turkey and Sweet Potato Casserole (44)	Soft Chocolate Sponge Cake Puree (69)
4	Apple, Raspberry with Vanilla Baby Food Puree (29)	Easy Creamy Vegetable Soup (35)	Pureed Lentil and Spinach Dahl (45)	Puréed Rice Pudding (69)
5	Yogurt Nog Smoothie (30)	Velvety Butternut and Cauliflower Soup (36)	Pureed Chickpea and Carrot Stew (45)	Puréed Apple Crumble (70)
6	Honey Shake (31)	Moroccan Pureed Vegetable Soup (36)	Pureed Eggplant and Tomato Ragout (46)	Fresh Banana Curd Puree (70)
7	Nutty Chocolate Milkshake (32)	Puree of Winter Vegetable Soup (37)	Pureed Zucchini and Basil Soup (46)	Strawberry Mousse Puree (70)
8	Spiced Pear Oat Baby Food Puree (26)	Broccoli and Spinach Pureed Soup (37)	Pureed Cauliflower and Cheese Bake (47)	Mango Panna Cotta Puree (71)
9	Roasted Blueberry + Cinnamon Baby Food Puree (28)	Carrot and Ginger Pureed Soup (38)	Pureed Green Bean and Potato Medley (47)	Peanut Butter Mousse Puree (71)
10	Banana + Coconut Milk + Cinnamon Baby Food Puree (30)	Potato and Leek Pureed Soup (38)	Pureed Carrot and Pea Side Dish (48)	Peach Mousse Puree (71)
11	Blackberry + Kale + Apple Baby Food Puree (29)	Roasted Red Pepper and Tomato Puree (39)	Pureed Butternut Squash and Apple Mash (48)	Homemade Vanilla Pudding (71)
12	Oats, Spinach, and Avocado Baby Food Puree (27)	Sweet Potato and Apple Puree (39)	Pureed Sweet Corn and Potato Chowder (48)	Passion Fruit Pudding Cake (72)
13	Vanilla Milkshake (32)	Creamy Mushroom Soup Puree (39)	Pureed Spinach and Potato Gratin (49)	Easy Milk Pudding (72)
14	Hawaiian Shake (30)	Parsnip and Celery Root Puree (40)	Pureed Root Vegetable Medley (49)	Simple Chocolate Mousse Puree (72)

15	Malted Milk Smoothie (31)	Roasted Pumpkin and Sage Puree (40)	Pureed Chicken Curry with Coconut Milk (54)	Raspberry Sorbet Puree (73)
16	3 Berry + Apple Baby Food Puree (27)	Cauliflower and White Bean Puree (41)	Pureed Turkey and Broccoli Bake (55)	Ube Halaya Puree (73)
17	Apple + Mint with Cottage Cheese Baby Food Puree (30)	Pea and Mint Pureed Soup (41)	Pureed Tuna and Sweet Corn Chowder (56)	Pots de Crème Puree (73)
18	Peach, Mango + Carrot Baby Food Puree (28)	Lentil and Carrot Puree (41)	Pureed Shrimp and Pumpkin Soup (56)	Creamy Mango Pudding (74)
19	Cinnamon Roll Breakfast Smoothie (26)	Butternut Squash and Coconut Milk Puree (42)	Pureed Chickpea and Carrot Stew (57)	Coconut Rice Pudding Puree (74)
20	Roasted Banana + Apple with Cinnamon Baby Food Puree (28)	Creamy Asparagus Puree (42)	Pureed Beef and Barley Soup (57)	Lemon Custard Puree (74)
21	Apple, Raspberry with Vanilla Baby Food Puree (29)	Pureed Chicken and Vegetable Stew (43)	Pureed Eggplant and Lentil Ragout (58)	Puréed Sticky Toffee Pudding (68)
22	Blackberry + Kale + Apple Baby Food Puree (29)	Pureed Beef and Root Vegetable Mash (43)	Pureed Greek Yogurt and Cucumber Dip (58)	Puréed Banoffee Pie (68)
23	Banana + Coconut Milk + Cinnamon Baby Food Puree (30)	Pureed Turkey and Sweet Potato Casserole (44)	Pureed Ham and Cheese Soup (59)	Soft Chocolate Sponge Cake Puree (69)
24	Yogurt Nog Smoothie (30)	Creamy Salmon and Potato Puree (44)	Pureed Lentil and Carrot Curry (52)	Puréed Rice Pudding (69)
25	Honey Shake (31)	Pureed Lentil and Spinach Dahl (45)	Creamy Pureed Cottage Cheese and Peas (53)	Puréed Apple Crumble (70)
26	Nutty Chocolate Milkshake (32)	Pureed Chickpea and Carrot Stew (45)	Pureed Egg and Cheese Casserole (53)	Fresh Banana Curd Puree (70)
27	Mango + Kale Baby Food Puree with Ginger (27)	Pureed Eggplant and Tomato Ragout (46)	Pureed White Fish and Potato Blend (53)	Strawberry Mousse Puree (70)
28	Roasted Pear + Date Baby Food Puree (28)	Pureed Zucchini and Basil Soup (46)	Pureed Black Bean and Quinoa Mash (54)	Mango Panna Cotta Puree (71)
29	Cinnamon Roll Breakfast Smoothie (26)	Pureed Cauliflower and Cheese Bake (47)	Pureed Chicken Curry with Coconut Milk (54)	Peanut Butter Mousse Puree (71)
30	Spiced Pear Oat Baby Food Puree (26)	Pureed Green Bean and Potato Medley (47)	Pureed Turkey and Broccoli Bake (55)	Peach Mousse Puree (71)
31	Oats, Spinach, and Avocado Baby Food Puree (27)	Pureed Carrot and Pea Side Dish (48)	Pureed Tuna and Sweet Corn Chowder (56)	Homemade Vanilla Pudding (71)
32	Roasted Blueberry + Cinnamon Baby Food Puree	Pureed Butternut Squash	Pureed Shrimp and	Passion Fruit Pudding

	(28)	and Apple Mash (48)	Pumpkin Soup (56)	Cake (72)
33	Apple + Mint with Cottage Cheese Baby Food Puree (30)	Pureed Sweet Corn and Potato Chowder (48)	Pureed Chickpea and Carrot Stew (57)	Easy Milk Pudding (72)
34	Banana + Coconut Milk + Cinnamon Baby Food Puree (30)	Pureed Spinach and Potato Gratin (49)	Pureed Beef and Barley Soup (57)	Simple Chocolate Mousse Puree (72)
35	Yogurt Nog Smoothie (30)	Pureed Root Vegetable Medley (49)	Pureed Eggplant and Lentil Ragout (58)	Raspberry Sorbet Puree (73)
36	Hawaiian Shake (30)	Pureed Chicken and Vegetable Medley (50)	Pureed Greek Yogurt and Cucumber Dip (58)	Ube Halaya Puree (73)
37	Honey Shake (31)	Creamy Pureed Turkey and Sweet Potato (50)	Pureed Ham and Cheese Soup (59)	Pots de Crème Puree (73)
38	Malted Milk Smoothie (31)	Pureed Salmon and Cauliflower Mash (51)	Pureed Chicken Curry with Coconut Milk (54)	Creamy Mango Pudding (74)
39	Nutty Chocolate Milkshake (32)	High-Protein Tofu and Spinach Puree (51)	Pureed Turkey and Broccoli Bake (55)	Coconut Rice Pudding Puree (74)
40	Vanilla Milkshake (32)	Pureed Beef and Root Vegetable Stew (52)	Pureed Tuna and Sweet Corn Chowder (56)	Lemon Custard Puree (74)
41	3 Berry + Apple Baby Food Puree (27)	Creamy Sweet Potato and Coconut Puree (60)	Roasted Cauliflower and Garlic Puree (60)	Puréed Sticky Toffee Pudding (68)
42	Apple, Raspberry with Vanilla Baby Food Puree (29)	Butternut Squash and Sage Puree (61)	Green Pea and Mint Puree (61)	Puréed Banoffee Pie (68)
43	Oats, Spinach, and Avocado Baby Food Puree (27)	Carrot and Ginger Puree (61)	Spinach and Avocado Puree (62)	Soft Chocolate Sponge Cake Puree (69)
44	Mango + Kale Baby Food Puree with Ginger (27)	Parsnip and Apple Puree (62)	Zucchini and Basil Puree (62)	Puréed Rice Pudding (69)
45	Cinnamon Roll Breakfast Smoothie (26)	Broccoli and Cauliflower Mash (63)	Pumpkin and Cinnamon Puree (63)	Puréed Apple Crumble (70)

Conclusion

As we reach the conclusion of this comprehensive guide, it is clear that embracing a pureed diet does not mean sacrificing flavor, nutrition, or the joy of eating. This book has been thoughtfully crafted to transform what can often be perceived as a limitation into a realm of culinary creativity, nourishment, and comfort. Whether you or your loved one face challenges with chewing, swallowing, or digestion, the recipes and techniques shared here empower you to prepare meals that are not only safe and appropriate but also delicious and visually appealing.

Pureed foods, by nature, are smooth and homogenous in texture, designed to be easily consumed without the need for chewing. Yet, as we have explored, true art lies in balancing texture and flavor to create meals that delight the palate and satisfy nutritional needs. The right texture-smooth but not sticky or lumpy-combined with vibrant colors, fresh herbs, and carefully chosen spices, can elevate pureed dishes beyond mere sustenance to an enjoyable dining experience.

Throughout this book, we have emphasized the importance of using quality kitchen tools like food processors and blenders to achieve perfect consistency, as well as creative presentation methods such as molds and piping techniques to enhance the appeal of pureed meals. We have also highlighted the significance of tailoring recipes to accommodate dietary restrictions, allergies, and personal preferences, ensuring that every meal supports health and well-being.

Nutrition remains at the heart of this journey. By incorporating a diverse range of fruits, vegetables, proteins, and whole grains, these recipes provide balanced nourishment essential for healing, energy, and vitality. From high-protein purees to allergy-friendly and vegan options, this guide offers something for everyone, making it a valuable resource for caregivers, healthcare professionals, and individuals alike.

Importantly, this book encourages a mindset shift: pureed diets are not a compromise but an opportunity to explore new flavors, textures, and presentations that honor the dignity and enjoyment of eating. With patience, creativity, and the knowledge shared here, you can bring joy back to mealtimes, fostering connection and comfort through food.

We hope this guide inspires you to embrace pureed cooking with confidence and passion, transforming each meal into a moment of care and celebration. Remember, food is more than fuel-it is love, culture, and life itself, and even in pureed form, it can nourish the body and soul alike.

Note

Made in the USA
Columbia, SC
01 July 2025

60188643R00057